Psychiatry
for the
House Officer
Second Edition

BOOKS IN THE HOUSE OFFICER SERIES

Psychiatry for the House Officer

Second Edition

David A. Tomb, M.D.
Department of Psychiatry
University of Utah School of Medicine
Salt Lake City, Utah

WILLIAMS & WILKINS
Baltimore • London • Los Angeles • Sydney

Editor: James L. Sangston
Associate Editor: Joseph E. Seitz
Design: James R. Mulligan
Illustration Planning: Joseph Cummings
Production: Raymond E. Reter

Copyright ©, 1984
Williams & Wilkins
428 East Preston Street
Baltimore, MD 21202, U.S.A.

Accurate indications, adverse reactions, and dosage schedules for drugs are provided in this book, but it is possible that they may change. The reader is urged to review the package information data of the manufacturers of the medications mentioned.

Made in the United States of America

First Edition, 1981
 Reprinted 1982, 1983, 1984

Library of Congress Cataloging in Publication Data

Main entry under title:

Tomb, David A.
 Psychiatry for the house officer.
 Includes bibliographies and index.
 1. Psychiatry—Handbooks, manuals, etc. 2. Mental illness—Handbooks, manuals, etc. 3. Psychological manifestations of general diseases—Handbooks, manuals, etc. I. Title. [DNLM: 1. Mental Disorders—handbooks. WM 34 T656p]
RC456.T65   1984   616.89   84-7404
ISBN 0-683-08338-4

Composed and printed at the
Waverly Press, Inc.   86 87 88 89   10 9 8 7 6 5 4

To my wife Jane and my daughter Collin
for time lost

Foreword

This book encompasses in distilled form much of what is clinically relevant in the field of modern psychiatry. A much larger book would have been easier to write. Condensing the vast amount of material covered in a readable, information-packed volume does credit to Dr. Tomb.

This volume should serve as an important resource for the medical student, the non-psychiatric house officer, and the practicing non-psychiatrist. It will be a very useful beginning text, in addition, for the psychiatric house officer since it discusses in a very few pages an enormous amount of specific medical/psychiatric information. For that reason it is suited admirably as a board review source.

This short text leaves the reader little doubt that the discipline of psychiatry has an extensive and well-founded body of "facts" which needs to be mastered if a physician is to treat his patients adequately. Dr. Tomb also clearly discusses the large number of patients with psychiatric problems who first present to the non-psychiatric physician and who need to be recognized and treated.

I expect that Psychiatry for the House Officer will become justifiably popular since it fills a need for a concise, factual volume for house officers and a trustworthy reference for busy practicing physicians.

Bernard I. Grosser, MD

David A. Tomb, MD, an adult and child psychiatrist,
is a faculty member in the Department of Psychiatry
of the University of Utah School of Medicine. He
was formerly the Clinical Director of the Utah
State Hospital and the Director of Psychiatric
Inpatient Services at the University of Utah
Medical Center. He was graduated from the College
of Wooster and the Pennsylvania State University
Medical School. He is active in teaching and in
the practice of adult and child psychiatry.

With a Foreword by Bernard I. Grosser, MD

Bernard I. Grosser, MD, is the chairman of the
Department of Psychiatry of the University of Utah
School of Medicine and is the Director of Clinical
Services at the University of Utah Medical Center.
He has been an active member of the International
Society for Psychoneuroendocrinology and has
published widely in the field of neuroendocrinology.

Preface to the Second Edition

Advances during the four years since publication of the first edition of this book have further clarified the various DSM-III disorders, suggested the proper clinical use of diagnostic tools such as the Dexamethasone Suppression Test (DST) and measures of urinary MHPG, and expanded the concepts of conditions such as bulimia and multiple personality. New psychopharmacologic agents have become available, as have refined psychotherapeutic techniques. In addition, psychiatry has experienced many other important refinements of fact and theory.

This new edition reflects these changes. I have made the information current and expanded and updated the references in each chapter. Throughout, I have attempted to capsulize the increasingly complex subject of modern psychiatry as briefly as possible. Spend the time thus saved with the real teachers: your patients.

David A. Tomb, MD
1984

Preface to the First Edition

Psychiatry is a field in ferment. There is much new information and there are several expanding areas of rapidly increasing sophistication. This book is an effort to present that information in a condensed but usable form. Since this book is designed for the non-psychiatric physician as well as the psychiatric resident, I have made an effort to emphasize medical/psychiatric correlations where they occur.

Throughout this book I have attempted to describe psychiatry in terms of the new official nomenclature, DSM-III, and each diagnosis is keyed to the identical diagnosis in DSM-III, both by number and page. To that extent, this book can also serve as an aid to diagnosis.

Although not meant to be comprehensive, I hope this manual gives a sense of the scope of current psychiatric knowledge. Psychiatry remains part art, part science. This book emphasizes the science while recognizing that it is frequently the art that heals. Armed with a core of facts, I hope that physicians will feel thoroughly comfortable when dealing with psychiatric patients, for that's where the action really is.

David A. Tomb, MD

Acknowledgments

This manual would have been quite different without
the help of those who read the various parts of it. I
particularly want to thank those physicians who had the
temerity to read the majority of the manuscript in rough
form: Doctors W. McMahon and L. King. I also am grateful
to the following people for reading and criticizing
selected chapters: Doctors P. Wender, B. Grosser, and L.
Schmidt. Also my thanks go to those psychiatric residents
who did battle with various chapters at various times.

Contents

Chapter 1

Psychiatric Classification

Psychiatric diagnosis has long been criticized as ambiguous and unreliable. Some diagnostic categories have been based on subjective, unverifiable intrapsychic phenomena, while others have been heterogeneously broad.

There are two responses to the familiar complaint of "why bother" using such imprecise tools.

1. There is a new, more reliable official classification scheme (DSM-III) which, although of uncertain validity, allows a more testable, scientific approach to mental disorders. This classification shall be used throughout this manual.
2. New and effective treatments for certain conditions (eg, some depressions, mania) make diagnostic specificity essential.

DSM-III

1980 saw the introduction of an innovative official psychiatric classification scheme in the USA: the 3rd edition of the Diagnostic and Statistical Manual of Mental Disorders (DSM-III). This scheme asserts that there are a limited number of identifiable psychiatric disorders. DSM-III contains specific diagnostic criteria for each diagnosis. One matches facts from a particular patient's history and clinical presentation with those criteria from a likely diagnosis and if an adequate number are met, that diagnosis should be made. Each disorder has a unique set of diagnostic criteria. Multiple diagnoses are permitted and there are several specific categories of "atypical" disorders which allow for placement of the (often many) patients who have unusual presentations.

For example: A patient who (1) has been having auditory hallucinations which (2) have impaired his social relations and functioning at work (3) for at least 6 months and who is without signs of (4) a Major Affective Disorder or (5) an Organic Mental Disorder must be given the diagnosis of Schizophrenic Disorder. If the patient also has (6) a flat, incongruous, or silly affect and (7) frequent or constant incoherence, an additional diagnosis of Disorganized subtype must be made.

MULTIAXIAL CLASSIFICATION:

In addition to the operationally defined criteria, DSM-III also introduces a multiaxial system of classification. A patient is not fully classified until he is coded on each of five axes (although only the first three axes are needed for an official diagnosis):

- Axis   I: The psychiatric syndrome (example above).
- Axis II: A personality disorder in adults; a
              Developmental Deviation in children (none
              may be present).
- Axis III: Physical disorders (none may be present).
- Axis IV: A severity rating of psychosocial stress during
              the past year.
- Axis   V: A measure of the highest functioning reached
              over the preceding year.

The specific rating scales for each axis are included in the text of DSM-III.

FUNDAMENTAL PSYCHIATRIC CONCEPTS

Psychiatric pathology is organized into several broad categories.

PSYCHOSIS: A general term referring to a major mental disorder having a marked impairment of:

- a sense of reality, and
- the ability to communicate, and/or
- emotional awareness and control, and/or
- cognitive abilities

which lead (1) to an inability to maintain interpersonal relations and (2) to compromised daily functioning. The principle types of psychotic disorders are:

1. Schizophrenic, Paranoid, and Schizoaffective
      Disorders
2. Schizophreniform Disorder and Brief Reactive
      Psychosis
3. Some Major Affective Disorders
4. Severe Organic Brain Syndromes

Some of these have known organic causes; some do not (ie, the functional psychoses).

PERSONALITY DISORDER: A long-standing, maladaptive personality trait of little concern to the patient but which causes impaired life adjustment.

NEUROSES: A theoretical grouping of diverse, chronic, non-psychotic, uncomfortable psychiatric conditions based on presumed unresolved intrapsychic conflicts (eg, phobias, hypochondriasis, Hysterical Neurosis).

REFERENCES

1. American Psychiatric Association Task Force on Nomenclature and Statistics: Diagnostic and Statistical Manual of Mental Disorders, 3rd ed. (DSM-III). American Psychiatric Association, Washington, D.C., 1980.
2. Andreasen NC, Hoenk PR: The predictive value of adjustment disorders: a follow-up study. Am J Psychiat 139:584, 1982.
3. Fleck S: A holistic approach to family typology and the axes of DSM-III. Arch Gen Psychiat 40:901, 1983.
4. Fox HA: The DSM-III concept of organic brain syndrome. Brit J Psychiat 142:419, 1983.
5. Longabaugh R, Fowler DR, Stout R, Kriebel G: Validation of a problem-focused nomenclature. Arch Gen Psychiat 40:453, 1983.
6. Mellsop G, Varghese F, Joshua S, Hicks A: The reliability of axis II of DSM-III. Am J Psychiat 139:1360, 1982.
7. Mezzich JE, Coffman GA, Goodpastor SM: A format for DSM-III diagnostic formulation: experience with 1,111 consecutive patients. Am J Psychiat 139:591, 1982.
8. Spitzer RL, Williams JBW, Skodol AE: DSM-III: The major achievements and an overview. Am J Psychiat 137:151, 1980.

Chapter 2

Assessment

A psychiatric evaluation helps (1) make a diagnosis, (2) estimate the severity of the patient's condition, (3) decide on an initial course of action, (4) develop a relationship with the patient, (5) assemble a dynamic understanding of the patient, and (6) engage the patient in psychotherapy. Some (primarily analytically oriented) psychiatrists argue that the most reliable understanding of a patient results from an open-ended interview in which the course of the interview is directed by the patient's conscious and unconscious concerns. An alternate form of interview, and one encouraged by the requirements of DSM-III, requires a structured format that demands precise historical and descriptive information and the answers to specific questions. Which technique produces a fuller understanding of the patient remains unresolved, yet modern diagnosis requires the structured form described below.

A thorough evaluation of a psychiatric patient consists of a psychiatric history, mental status examination, complete physical examination, laboratory screening evaluation, and selected psychological and laboratory tests when indicated. The history and mental status are usually obtained during the initial interview.

More is required in this process than merely collecting facts. The interviewer seeks useful information from the facts of the history and mental status examination, but also from the sequence in which the patient mentions things, the patient's interpersonal style, and the patient's non-verbal communication. Because there is so much information available from the patient outside the formal part of the interview, it is essential to avoid structuring the interview too early. Early on, allow the patient to express his concerns and find out his reason for coming for help (Why now?). Be supportive and encouraging - develop a rapport with the patient and try to get an empathic understanding of his distress. Help allay

anxiety, if present. Be patient, friendly, and receptive
if the patient is quiet. If he rambles, you may have to
impose a structure earlier. Develop a qualitative sense
for the patient's impairment. Is he likely to be
aggressive? Suicidal? In need of hospitalization?

If skillfully conducted, much of the information
required by the history and mental status exam may be
obtained unobtrusively during this period. Also, as the
interview proceeds, it is possible to more clearly identify
and narrow what is relevant so that the formal demand for
specific information may be minimal. However, some such
information is almost always required (eg, data to satisfy
DSM-III diagnostic criteria, family psychiatric history, or
mental status responses to rule out organicity or loss of
abstracting ability) so at times during the interview
mentally review what is missing and save time towards the
end to pursue it by direct questioning. The transition to
a more formal style of interviewing can be smooth if
rapport has been developed beforehand.

PSYCHIATRIC HISTORY

IDENTIFICATION OF THE PATIENT:

1. Name, age, birth date, marital status and children,
   race, religion, occupation, education, social class,
   handicaps, etc.
2. Identification of informants (if not the patient). Mood
   and apparent biases of informants.
3. Estimate of the reliability of the information.

CHIEF COMPLAINT:

Usually a verbatim statement of "what the problem is."
Does it differ significantly from the reports of those who
accompany the patient?

PRESENT ILLNESS:

Usually the focus of the interview. Get the patient's
description of and feelings about his illness. Establish
chronological order of symptoms and treatments. Has the
patient noticed any other changes in himself? Major life
changes during this time? Stresses and conflicts? Any
secondary gain identifiable? Past psychiatric history? -
particularly diagnosis and severity of illness; types of
treatment; drug use.

PAST PERSONAL HISTORY:

Birth and early development - relatives may be a source
of information: Mother's pregnancy and delivery;
prematurity? planned pregnancy? Get estimate of
temperament and behavior problems. Psychophysiological problems?

Childhood: Personality traits, behavior problems, social
relationships, school adjustment, family relationships
and stability.

Social history: What kind of interpersonal relationships can the patient make? - has he been a loner?
follower? leader? What kind of group activities in
the past and in the present? Who are the people
important to him now? in the past? What was his
premorbid personality? Military history?

Marriage: At what age? How many times? Relationship
patterns within the marriage? Number of children and
attitude toward them?

Education: Highest grade attained? Specific academic
difficulties? Behavior problems? Social problems?

Occupational history: Should be fairly detailed with
concentration on job changes, length of time jobs have
been held, best job obtained and when. Social relations
on job; with boss? with workers? How does job
compare with ambition? with family expectations?

Sexual history: Sexual orientation? Psychosexual
problems or deviant behavior? Feelings about sex?

FAMILY HISTORY:

Who lives in the home? - patient should describe them
and describe his relationship with them. Description of
patient's family of origin and his role in it. Upwardly
mobile family? Get detailed description of psychiatric
(and medical) illnesses in family members.

MEDICAL HISTORY:

Current and past medical problems and treatments.

CURRENT SOCIAL SITUATION:

Personal living situation, income? Social
environment? Estimated current marital and family
stability and happiness?

MENTAL STATUS EXAMINATION

A mental status examination is a systematic documen-
tation of the quality of mental functioning at the time of

the interview. It both helps with current diagnosis and treatment planning and it serves as a baseline for future reference. Although much of the information sought in a mental status exam is obtained informally during other parts of the interview, it is usually necessary for the patient to answer a few formal questions if the interviewer is to learn the patient's abilities in each of the categories of mental functioning listed below. Upon concluding the mental status examination, estimate its reliability.

GENERAL PRESENTATION:

Appearance - overall impression of the patient:
attractive, unattractive, posture, clothes, grooming, healthy vs sickly, old looking vs young looking, angry, puzzled, frightened, ill-at-ease, apathetic, contemptuous, effeminate, masculine, etc.
General behavior: mannerisms, gestures, combative, psychomotor retardation, rigid, twitches, picking, clumsy, hand wringing, etc.
Attitude towards the examiner: cooperative, hostile, defensive, seductive, evasive, ingratiating, etc.

The psychotic patient may appear disheveled and bizarre with odd posturing (particularly catatonics) and grimacing. Some schizophrenics may stare and others look "blank." Paranoid patients may be hostile while hysterical patients often are seductive in manner and dress. Depressed patients may be nearly mute and display psychomotor retardation. Restlessness may suggest anxiety, drug withdrawal, mania, etc.

STATE OF CONSCIOUSNESS:

Is the patient alert (eg, normally aware of both internal and external stimuli) or is he hyperalert? Is the patient lethargic - eg, does he "drift off" or do his thoughts wander? The patient needs to be reasonably alert for the remainder of the exam to be reliable. The causes for decreased alertness are usually organic.

ATTENTION:

Can the patient pay attention for short periods of time (attend) without being distracted by minor stimuli? Can he attend for lengths of time (concentrate)? This ability is necessary if you are to assess higher level functions (ie, they may be intact but the patient can't demonstrate it due to lack of attention). Test attention by digit recall - eg, speak a series of numbers in a monotone and ask the patient to repeat them; begin with

three and increase by one with each successful trial; a
normal maximum response is 6 numbers repeated. Test
concentration by Random Letter Test - eg, tell patient to
note (by raising his finger) each time a certain letter is
mentioned and then read a long string of letters; most
people make very few errors. Defects in attention usually
are due to organic causes but may be caused by marked
anxiety or psychotic interruption of thoughts.

SPEECH:

Listen to the patient's speech. Is it loud, soft,
fast, slow, pressured, mute, etc? Does the patient speak
spontaneously? with good vocabulary? Does the patient
articulate with difficulty (dysarthria)?

Is there a deficiency in language - eg, aphasia? This
speech is usually identifiable by the experienced listener
(eg, patient tries to communicate but incorrect words are
chosen and grammatical errors made) but may be confused
with rambling psychotic speech. Manic patients often speak
loudly and rapidly; depressed patients are soft and slow.
Bizarre speech usually suggests a psychotic and/or organic
state.

ORIENTATION:

Check for person (name? age? when born?), place (What
place is this? What is your home address?), time (today's
date? day of the week? time? season?), and situation
(Why are you here?). Time sense is usually the first lost.
Major disorientation suggests organicity. Minor loss may
reflect temporary stress.

MOOD AND AFFECT:

Mood is a sustained emotional state - eg, depressed,
   euphoric, elevated, anxious, angry, irritable.
Affect is the patient's current emotional state - it is
   the state the interviewer can observe. Common
   abnormal affects include flat, blunted, and
   inappropriate.

Note whether the affect you observe is consistent with
the patient's expressed mood and congruent with his thought
content. Distinguish a depressed mood from an organically
caused apathy. The affective disorders most commonly
display alterations in mood but so do psychotic, anxiety
(eg, panic), and organic (eg, drug use) disorders.

FORM OF THOUGHT:

Does the patient's thinking make sense? Does one thought follow another logically or does the patient display circumstantiality (take forever to make his point; many unnecessary details - overinclusiveness), flight of ideas (rapidly jumping from idea to idea, but with understandable associations), evasiveness, loosening of associations (tangentiality - thoughts are unrelated but the patient seems unaware of this), perseveration (needless repetition of the same thought or phrase), or blocking (speech and train of thought is interrupted and picked up again a few moments or minutes later). Are answers to questions relevant? Ask the patient for his impressions of his own thoughts.

These abnormalities in thought process are most commonly associated with schizophrenic or affective disorders. None are pathognomonic but any major abnormality suggests a psychotic process.

THOUGHT CONTENT:

Check for: abnormal preoccupations and obsessions, excessive suspiciousness, phobias, rituals, hypochondriacal symptoms, deja vu experiences, depersonalization, delusions (fixed, false beliefs - characterize them as persecutory, of grandeur, of reference, of influence, unsystematized, etc). Always check for preoccupations about suicide or homicide.

Get at the presence of delusions by questions like: "Do you have any strong ideas other people don't share?; Are there things you think about a lot?"

Delusions usually suggest a functional psychotic disorder (most commonly schizophrenia) but other conditions may display them (eg, poorly systematized delusions in OBS). Obsessions may occur with psychosis but also are typical of obsessive compulsive disorder. Phobias characterize phobic disorders.

Is the patient unaware that he is ill or has abnormal thinking (lacks insight)? Does he have a generalized loss of ability for abstractive thinking (ie, concreteness)? Test for abstractive ability by:
1. Similarities: "What do these things have in common?"

        baseball - orange
            car - train
           desk - bookcase

        happy - sad
        horse - apple

2. Proverbs: "What do people mean when they say. . .?"

        When the cat's away, the mice will play.
        The proof of the pudding is in the eating.
        A golden hammer breaks an iron door.
        The tongue is the enemy of the neck.
        The hot coal burns, the cold one blackens.

Always correlate abstractive thinking with intelligence.
Concreteness in the face of normal intelligence is suggestive of a psychotic thought disorder (although this is
questioned - see Andreasen, 1977). Note any bizarre
responses to similarities or proverbs - are the answers
personalized? Are the answers vague because the patient is
aware of failing (eg, OBS) and is obfuscating?

PERCEPTIONS:

        Does the patient display misperceptions (draw wrong
conclusions from self-evident information)? Are there
illusions (misinterpretations of sensory stimuli - eg, a
shadow becomes a person) or hallucinations (note whether
auditory, visual, tactile, olfactory, etc)? Always
determine if hallucinations are accusatory, threatening, or
commanding. If not volunteered, get at the presence of
hallucinations by questions like: "Have you had the experience of walking down the street, hearing your name called,
and finding no one there? Have you had any mystical or
psychic experiences?"

        Illusions are most common in delirium but may also
occur in functional psychoses. Hallucinations occur in a
variety of conditions but most commonly in psychotic
disorders. Schizophrenia usually has auditory
hallucinations while visual hallucinations are more common
in organic conditions. Tactile hallucinations are frequent
in sedative-hypnotic and alcohol withdrawal states.

JUDGEMENT:

        An estimate of the patient's real life problem solving
skills is often difficult to make. Judgement is a complex
mental function which depends on maturation of the nervous
system (poor in children). The best indicator is usually
the patient's behavior, so history is very important. Some
sense of the patient's judgement can be obtained through
hypothetical examples: "What should you do if you find a
stamped, addressed letter? What should you do if you lose

a book belonging to a library?"

Judgement is regularly impaired in OBS, psychosis, and some retardation. Its assessment helps determine the patient's capacity for independent functioning.

MEMORY:

Test all three types of memory: remote, recent, and immediate (retention and recall).

Immediate:
  1. Digit repetition
  2. Ask patient to remember 3 objects and 3 words - ask for them after 5 minutes (they should be recalled).
  3. Ask the patient to count - stop him at 27 - (wait 1 minute) - tell him to continue counting - stop at 42 - (wait 3 minutes) - then continue counting.

Recent: Ask questions about the past 24 hours - eg, "How did you travel here? What was on the news last night?"

Remote: Personal - born? school? work? etc.
          Historical - name four presidents in this century; the dates of WW II; etc.

Recent and remote memory usually can be tested inconspicuously during the interview. Is the patient aware of his deficit? What is his attitude toward it? Loss of memory usually indicates an organic process unless it has some of the characteristics of the dissociative disorders (chapter 9).

Constructional ability is a sensitive test for early diffuse cortical damage. Draw a diamond and a 3-dimensional cube and have the patient copy them. Ask the patient to draw a flowerpot with a flower, or the face of a clock set at 2:45. Incomplete or very poorly done responses are suggestive of early organicity.

INTELLECTUAL FUNCTIONING:

Intelligence is a global function which can be estimated from the general tone and content of the interview as well as by the patient's fund of information and ability to perform calculations.

Fund of knowledge:

How many weeks in a year?
Name the last 6 presidents.

What does the liver do?
How far is it from Chicago to LA?
Why are light colored clothes cool?
Who wrote Remembrances of Things Past?
What causes rust?

How many nickels in $1.15.

Calculations:

serial 7's - "Take 100 and subtract 7 from it, then
    take 7 from the answer, etc."
serial 3's - eg, take 3 from 20, etc.
simple calculations - 2x3, 5x3, 4x9.

Calculation relies on functions other than intelligence including concentration and memory. If in doubt, ask
for formal IQ testing. Organic conditions may produce a
loss of intellectual functioning but psychoses seldom do
(as long as the patient can concentrate on the tests).

PSYCHOLOGICAL TESTS

Psychological testing is requested for occasional
psychiatric patients and may provide a useful enlargement
of the understanding of those patients. Although not
essential for most patients, testing may:

1. Help identify organic syndromes.
2. Help localize organic pathology.
3. Contribute to the identification of borderline psychotic
   states.
4. Provide a baseline of general and specific functioning.
5. Generally help with differential diagnosis among
   psychiatric conditions.

Talk to the psychologist. Describe what you are looking for. Ask for recommendations. Although most patients
receive a battery of tests, very specific questions may be
answered by only one test. Carefully integrate the psychologist's report with your own evaluation but do not allow
test results to supersede clinical judgement. Commonly
used tests for adults include:

Wechsler Adult Intelligence Scale (WAIS): A very useful
test. Although it does yield three separate IQ scores
(full-scale, verbal, and performance), a careful evaluation
of how the patient answered the 11 different subtests
within the WAIS provides clues to the presence of a thought

disorder, an attention or memory deficit, visual-motor impairment, etc.

Minnesota Multiphasic Personality Inventory (MMPI): This is a self-administered personality test which takes little of the therapist's time, produces a general description of the patient's personality characteristics, and even can be computer scored. Although a useful global description of the patient, do not stretch it too far diagnostically.

Bender-Gestalt Test: This test is easily administered - the patient draws nine specific geometric figures on a blank sheet of paper. Its greatest application is in detecting visual-motor impairment and organic deficits.

Rorschach Test: This is an unstructured projective test which asks the patient to "describe what he sees" in a series of ten standardized ink blots. Elaborate scoring systems exist which allow a skilled examiner to infer elements of the patient's personality functioning. It is used diagnostically to help identify psychoses and person- ality disorders. Its diagnostic validity has not been assured.

Thematic Apperception Test (TAT): This is a projective test similar to the Rorschach which draws conclusions from the patient's responses to a series of suggestive and ambiguous human figure drawings.

Draw-a-person Test: The patient is asked to draw a picture of a "person" and then a picture of a person of the opposite sex. The results are then interpreted by the examiner.

EEG

The EEG plays a useful supportive role in psychiatry. It is not definitive in any psychiatric condition but it does help rule in or out a diversity of conditions. Its primary use is in the differentiation between organic and functional conditions.

1. Epileptics (particularly temporal lobe epilepsy) often mimic psychiatric patients - the EEG helps differ- entiate (although 30% of epileptics have a normal tracing between attacks).
2. The patient who is confused and disoriented (delirium) due to organic factors usually has diffuse EEG slowing. A major exception is Alcohol Withdrawal Delirium (delirium tremens) which shows increased fast activity.
3. The patient who has Primary Degenerative Dementia (Alzheimer's Disease - 50% of demented patients)

usually has a normal EEG. Most reversible forms of
dementia produce abnormal tracings. The EEG of a
person with pseudodementia (eg, depression which
mimics dementia) is usually normal.
4. Drugs often alter the EEG - eg, sedative-hypnotics
    increase fast activity; major tranquilizers increase
    slow activity.
5. A variety of organic causes can produce bizarre behavior
    (eg, brain tumor, cerebral infarcts, cerebral trauma).
    A normal EEG does not rule out organic pathology but
    an abnormal tracing is suspicious.

Several populations of psychiatric patients have a
slightly increased frequency of nonspecific abnormalities
on the EEG - eg, schizophrenics (particularly catatonics)
and manic-depressives. Patients with Antisocial Personality Disorder have perhaps the highest frequency of abnormal
tracings - look for but don't over-read organic pathology
in these patients.

Many other biological measures may be helpful in
assessment, including CT scan, CBF measures, a variety of
laboratory tests, and PET scan (in research settings).

THE AMYTAL INTERVIEW

The administration of amobarbital (Amytal), thiopental
(Pentothal), pentobarbital (Nembutal) during an interview to
produce a sedated state has been used for many years both
diagnostically (Amytal interview) and therapeutically
(narcoanalysis). In spite of a long history of use, the
indications for and value of this technique are unclear.

The technique usually consists of administering a
total of 200-500 mg (occasionally more) of sodium
amobarbital IV at a rate of 25-50 mg/min. The interviewer
talks with the patient throughout administration and halts
the drug temporarily when the desired level of sedation is
attained (eg, appearance of lateral nystagmus for light
sedation; development of slurred speech for a deeper
state). Additional Amytal may be given if the interview is
lengthy.

In this sedated state some patients present a markedly
altered clinical picture which may be of diagnostic value.
Although opinion varies (Dysken et al, 1979), diagnostic
uses for the Amytal interview may include:

1. Evaluation of mute patients - Patients with catatonic
    schizophrenia often recover dramatically when sedated
    (although a thought disorder usually remains) but

return to the full catatonic state when the Amytal
wears off. This is very useful in differentiating
catatonia from marked psychomotor retardation in the
depressed patient (they show little improvement).
Patients mute for other reasons (eg, hysterical,
acute stress) may begin to talk under sedation.

2. Acute panic states - Patients immobilized by severe
   stress may talk about their concerns when sedated.
3. Organic vs functional differentiation - Patients who are
   confused, disoriented, or demented due to organic
   factors usually worsen with Amytal while clinically
   similar functional patients often clear temporarily.
4. Hysterical phenomena - Amnesias, fugues, and conversion
   disorders often are temporarily relieved by Amytal.
   Useful information may be obtained during this time -
   eg, the patient's name and address; the cause of the
   patient's anger.
5. The interview is less reliably useful with psychotic
   states (except for catatonic schizophrenia) although
   some patients may contribute information they wouldn't
   have otherwise.

Although helpful in confirming some diagnoses, the
Amytal interview also may contribute to the treatment of a
few patients by allowing them to confront and deal with
stressful or troubling experiences which they previously
had been reluctant or unable to face.

REFERENCES

1. Andreasen NC: Reliability and validity of proverb
   interpretation to assess mental status. Comp Psychiat
   18:465, 1977.
2. Dysken MW, Kooser JA, Haraszti JS, Davis JM: Clinical
   usefulness of sodium amobarbital interviewing. Arch Gen
   Psychiat 36:789, 1979.
3. Jacobs JW, Bernhard MR, Delgado A, Strain JJ: Screening
   for organic mental syndromes in the medically ill. Ann
   Int Med 86:40, 1977.
4. Katzman R, Brown T, Fuld P, Peck A, Schechter R,
   Schimmel H: Validation of a short orientation-memory-
   concentration test of cognitive impairment. Am J
   Psychiat 140:734, 1983.
5. Mackinnon RA, Michels R: The Psychiatric Interview in
   Clinical Practice. Philadelphia, WB Saunders, 1971.
6. Naples M, Hackett TP: The Amytal interview: history and
   current uses. Psychosomatics 19:98, 1978.
7. Perry JC, Jacobs D: Overview: clinical applications of
   the amytal interview in psychiatric emergency settings.
   Am J Psychiat 139:552, 1982.

8. Shagass C, Roemer RA, Straumanis JJ: Relationships between psychiatric diagnosis and some quantitative EEG variables. Arch Gen Psychiat 39:1423, 1982.
9. Strub RL, Black FW: The Mental Status Examination in Neurology. Philadelphia, FA Davis Co, 1977.
10. Sullivan HS: The Psychiatric Interview. New York, WW Norton and Co, 1954.

Chapter 3

Psychotic Disorders

"Psychosis" describes a degree of severity, not a specific disorder (see p 2). A psychotic patient has a grossly impaired sense of reality, often coupled with emotional and cognitive disabilities, which severely compromises his ability to function. He is likely to talk and act in a bizarre fashion, have hallucinations, or strongly hold ideas that are contrary to fact (delusions). He may be confused and disoriented.

This chapter covers all the major psychotic disorders - ie, conditions which <u>must</u> reach psychotic proportions at some time during their course (although the patients may be non-psychotic most of the time). Recognize that these are primarily descriptive groupings of clinical syndromes - <u>not</u> discrete diseases.

Schizophrenic Disorders:
    Disorganized type
    Catatonic type
    Paranoid type
    Undifferentiated type
    Residual type

Schizophreniform Disorder

Brief Reactive Psychosis

Schizoaffective Disorder

Paranoid Disorder
    Paranoia
    Shared Paranoid Disorder
    Acute Paranoid Disorder

Atypical Psychosis

DIFFERENTIAL DIAGNOSIS:

There are a variety of other conditions (psychiatric, medical, neurological) which occasionally can present with psychosis. There is a basic dichotomy which should be looked for. Some psychoses, like the conditions above, are functional (no certain organic, medical cause) while others are caused by physical factors (fever, trauma, infection, drugs, medical diseases, etc). Most of the functional conditions present with emotional and thinking disturbances in a patient with a clear sensorium while most of the organic psychoses have a degree of delirium (eg, clouding of consciousness, confusion, disorientation). Unfortunately, exceptions to either of these characterizations are frequent.

Since it is always important to identify organic conditions when they are present, obtain a complete history and physical on all psychotic patients, if possible. Suspect an organic etiology if:

- The patient presents with significant memory loss, confusion, disorientation, or clouding of consciousness.
- There is no personal or family history of serious psychiatric illness. A first episode of a functional psychosis is unusual after age 35.
- The patient has a serious medical illness or a chronic medical condition with periodic relapses.
- The psychosis has developed rapidly (eg, days) in a patient who previously had been functioning well.

Psychiatric conditions which may (but don't necessarily) reach psychotic proportions include:

1. Major Affective Disorder (see chapter 4) - look for the psychosis to coexist with and be dominated by an affective component (either manic or depressed) which preceded the development of the psychosis.
2. Organic Mental Disorders (see chapters 5 and 6) - possible etiologies include almost any type of serious medical illness (see also chapters 14 and 15).
3. Brief reactive psychoses may occur with stress in patients with personality disorders of the Histrionic, Borderline, Paranoid, and Schizotypal types. Some obsessive-compulsive persons at times may develop a psychosis if failing to control their environment.
4. Some acute panic or rage attacks may be of psychotic intensity - eg, acute homosexual panic; rage in the patient with an Explosive Disorder (see chapter 7).
5. A few psychotic conditions develop in childhood and

continue into the adult years - INFANTILE AUTISM
(DSM-III p 87, 299.0) and CHILDHOOD ONSET PERVASIVE
DEVELOPMENTAL DISORDER (DSM-III p 90, 299.9).
6. Psychotic states occasionally may be mimicked
   unconsciously or even "faked" - Factitious Disorder
   with Psychological Symptoms, Malingering.

SCHIZOPHRENIC DISORDERS

Schizophrenia is the most common psychotic disorder -
almost 1% of people worldwide develop it during their
lifetime; over 2 million persons are affected in the USA.
It occurs more frequently in urban populations and in lower
socioeconomic groups - probably due to a "downward drift"
(ie, poorly functional, unemployable persons end up in
marginal settings). Poor environments do not "cause" the
disorders, although they may make it more intractable.

The diagnosis of Schizophrenia has had a checkered
history. There have been numerous different ways to make
the diagnosis, which have thus represented numerous
different populations of patients. The current diagnostic
scheme (DSM-III) uses specific objective criteria to define
a set of Schizophrenic Disorders. Because there are no
pathognomonic findings, "schizophrenia" is a clinical
diagnosis which may represent a non-specific syndrome of
heterogeneous etiologies. However, biological, genetic,
and phenomenological information suggest that it is a valid
disorder(s). The five identified subtypes are also based
on clinical variables.

CLINICAL PRESENTATION:

While the nature of schizophrenia is uncertain, the
current clinical description and method of making the
diagnosis are more clear (DSM-III).

Most schizophrenics are psychotic for only a small
part of their lives. Typically they spend many years in a
residual phase during which time they display only minor
features of their illness. During these residual periods
the patients may be withdrawn, isolated, and "peculiar."
They usually are noticeable to others and may lose their
jobs or friends both because of their own lack of interest
and ability to perform and because they are behaving oddly.
Their thinking and speech is vague and is felt by others to
be odd and to "not quite make sense." They may be
convinced that they are different from others, feel that
they have special powers and sensitivities, and have
"mystical" or "psychic" experiences. Their personal

appearance and manners deteriorate and they may display affect which is blunted, flat, or inappropriate. They are frequently anhedonic (unable to experience pleasure). Often this deterioration merely represents a gradual worsening of a condition the patient has displayed for many years - the first psychotic episode may have been preceded by a similar period of eccentric thinking and behavior (prodromal phase).

A "prepsychotic personality" is seen in some chronic schizophrenics and is characterized by social withdrawal, social awkwardness, and marked shyness in a youth who has difficulty in school in spite of a normal IQ (Kendler et al, 1982; Parnas et al, 1982). An equally common pattern is involvement in minor antisocial activities in the year or two prior to the initial psychotic episode. Many of these patients have been diagnosed previously as having a Schizoid, Borderline, Antisocial, or Schizotypal Personality Disorder. It is only when they develop their first psychotic episode (normally in their teens and early 20's (men) or 20's and early 30's (women); a first "breakdown" after age 40 is unusual) that the diagnosis is changed to schizophrenia. Often a presumed precipitating stress can be identified. The typical acute psychosis displays a variable mixture of several of the following symptoms.

Disturbance of Thought Form: These patients usually have a formal thought disorder - ie, their thinking is frequently incomprehensible to others and appears illogical. Characteristics include:

Loosening of associations (tangential associations) - Patient's ideas are disconnected. He may jump obliviously from topic to unconnected topic, confusing the listener. When this occurs frequently (eg, in midsentence), the speech is often incoherent.
Overinclusiveness - Patient continually may disrupt the flow of his thoughts by including irrelevant information.
Neologisms - Patient coins new words (may have a symbolic meaning for him).
Blocking - Speech is halted (often in midsentence) and then picked up a moment (or minutes) later, usually at another place. This may represent the patient's ideas being interrupted by intrusive thoughts (eg, hallucinations). These patients are often very distractible and have a short attention span.
Clanging - The patient chooses his next words and themes based on the sound of the words he is using rather than the thought content. Usually he rhymes

a primary word in one sentence with a word in the
preceding sentence.

Echolalia - Patient repeats words or phrases in a
musical or singsong fashion but without an apparent
effort to communicate.

Concreteness - Patient of normal or above average IQ
thinks in abstract terms poorly.

Poverty of speech content - Patient may talk a lot and
say very little.

Disturbance of Thought Content: Delusions (fixed, false
beliefs - particularly ideas that are beyond
credibility and are not modified in spite of clear
evidence to the contrary) are common in most serious
mental disorders, but some specific forms of delusional
thought are particularly frequent in schizophrenia.
The more acute the psychosis, the more likely the
delusion is to be disorganized and nonsystematized.

Bizarre, confused delusions

Persecutory delusions - particularly nonsystematic
types.

Delusions of grandeur

Delusions of influence - patient believes that he can
control events through telepathy.

Delusions of reference - Patient is convinced that
there are "meanings" behind events and people's
actions which are directed specifically toward him.

Many schizophrenic patients display lack of insight -
ie, the patient is unaware of his own illness or of his
need for treatment, even though his disorder is evident
to others.

Disturbance of Perception: Most common are hallucinations,
usually auditory but also visual, olfactory, and
tactile. The auditory hallucinations (most often
voices - one or several) may include a running
commentary about the patient and events, derogatory or
threatening comments made to the patient, or direct
orders to the patient (command hallucinations). The
voices may be perceived as coming from outside or
inside the patient's head and occasionally the patient
may hear his own thoughts spoken aloud (often to his
shame or embarrassment). The voices are quite "real"
to the patient, except in the early phases of the
psychosis.

These patients may also have illusions, depersonal-
izations, derealizations, and a hallucinatory sense of
bodily change.

<u>Disturbance of Emotions</u>: Acutely psychotic patients may display any emotion and may switch from one to another in a surprisingly short span of time. Two frequent (but not pathognomonic) underlying affects are:

<u>Blunted or flat affect</u> - The patient expresses very little emotion, even when it is appropriate to·do so. He appears to be without warmth.

<u>Inappropriate affect</u> - The affect may be intense but it is inconsistent with the patient's thoughts or speech.

<u>Disturbance of Behavior</u>: Many different bizarre and inappropriate behaviors may be seen including strange grimacing and posturing, ritual behavior, excessive silliness, aggressiveness, and some sexual inappropriateness.

An acute psychotic attack can last weeks or months (occasionally years). Many patients have recurrences of the active phase periodically throughout their lives, typically separated by months or years. During the intervening periods, patients usually present residual symptoms (often with the degree of impairment gradually increasing over the years), however a few patients are symptom-free between acute episodes. Many schizophrenic patients in remission display early signs of a developing relapse (Herz and Melville, 1980) - always look for them. These early signs include increasing restlessness and nervousness, loss of appetite, mild depression and anhedonia, insomnia, and trouble concentrating.

<u>CLASSIFICATION</u>:

To be considered schizophrenic, a patient must (DSM-III, p 188)

1. have had at least <u>6 months</u> of
2. sufficiently <u>deteriorated</u> occupational, interpersonal, and self-supportive functioning at some time in the past,
3. with an onset <u>before 45 years</u> of age,
4. must have been <u>actively psychotic</u> in a characteristic fashion during at least part of that period,
5. must currently show some <u>signs of illness</u>, and
6. must not be able to account for the symptoms by the presence of a Major Affective Disorder, Organic Mental Disorder, or Mental Retardation.

All schizophrenic patients <u>must</u> be classed as one of five recognized subtypes which describe the most frequently occurring behavioral manifestations of the illness. There have been numerous subclassifications of schizophrenia in the past, all unsatisfactory, and the current divisions share some of those deficiencies. Although genetic data suggests that schizophrenia is a stable diagnosis, there is no comparable information for the subtypes. Symptomatically, they tend to overlap and the diagnosis can shift from one to another with time (either during one episode or in a subsequent episode). Finally, over the years, the clinical presentations of many patients tend to converge towards a common picture of interpersonal withdrawal, flattened affect, idiosyncratic thinking, and impaired social and personal functioning.

DISORGANIZED TYPE (DSM-III p 190, 295.1): The patient has (1) blunted, silly, or inappropriate affect, (2) frequent incoherence, and (3) no systematized delusions. Grimacing and bizarre mannerisms are common.

CATATONIC TYPE (DSM-III p 190, 295.2): The patient may have any one (or a combination) of several forms of catatonia.

1. Catatonic stupor or mutism - Patient does not appreciably respond to his environment or the people in it. In spite of appearances, these patients are often thoroughly aware of what is going on around them.
2. Catatonic negativism - Patient resists all directions or physical attempts to move him.
3. Catatonic rigidity - Patient is physically rigid.
4. Catatonic posturing - Patient assumes bizarre or unusual postures.
5. Catatonic excitement - Patient is extremely (eg, wildly) active and excited. May be life-threatening (eg, due to exhaustion).

PARANOID TYPE (DSM-III p 191, 295.3): This is the most stable subtype over time and usually develops later than other forms of schizophrenia. The patient must display one or more symptoms including (1) persecutory delusions, (2) grandiose delusions, (3) delusional jealousy, and (4) persecutory or grandiose hallucinations. These patients are often uncooperative and difficult to deal with and may be aggressive, angry, or fearful.

UNDIFFERENTIATED TYPE (DSM-III p 191, 295.9): The patient has prominent hallucinations, delusions, and other evidences of active psychosis (eg, confusion, incoherence) but without the more specific features of the preceding three categories.

RESIDUAL TYPE (DSM-III p 192, 295.6): The patient is in remission from active psychosis but displays symptoms of the residual phase (eg, social withdrawal, flat or inappropriate affect, eccentric behavior, loosening of associations and illogical thinking).

PROGNOSIS:

Schizophrenia is a chronic disorder. A person gradually may become more withdrawn, "eccentric," and non-functional over many years. Some patients may experience low-level delusions and hallucinations indefinitely. Many of the more dramatic and acute symptoms disappear with time but the patient ends up chronically needing sheltered living or spending years in mental hospitals. Involvement with the law for misdemeanors is common (eg, vagrancy, disturbing the peace). A few patients become markedly demented. Overall life expectancy is shortened - primarily due to accidents, suicide, and an inability of the patients to care for themselves.

This pattern has exceptions. Psychiatrists have long distinguished between process schizophrenia (slowly developing; chronic, deteriorating course) and reactive schizophrenia (rapid onset; relatively good prognosis). Clinical characteristics which suggest a better prognosis include:

1. A rapid onset of the active psychotic symptoms.
2. An onset after age 30.
3. Good premorbid social and occupational functioning. Past performance remains the best predictor of future performance.
4. Marked confusion and emotional features during the acute episode (some question this - eg, Gift et al, 1980).
5. A probable precipitating stress to the acute psychosis.
6. No family history of schizophrenia.

It may be that these are two etiologically (and biologically?) distinct disorders. Although there is great variability, Disorganized Type generally has the worst prognosis while Paranoid Type (and some catatonics) have the best. The patient's prognosis is worsened if he abuses drugs or if he lives in a family setting overtly hostile to him.

A common phenomenon among schizophrenics (25-50% of patients) recovering from an acute episode is a major

depression during the months following improvement
(postpsychotic depression - see Mandel et al, 1982).
Although treatment resistant, psychotherapy (Seeman and
McGee, 1982) and antidepressant medication may be useful
(lithium may also help - see VanKammen et al, 1980). Watch
for it - suicide rate is increased in this population.
Don't overdiagnose - some of these patients may have a
medication induced akinesia mimicking depression (Van
Putten et al, 1978).

BIOLOGY OF SCHIZOPHRENIA:

No pathognomonic structural or functional abnormality
has been found in schizophrenics, however, numerous
intriguing abnormalities exist (and have been replicated,
as well as contested) in subpopulations of patients:
frontal concentrations of neuropeptides, increased platelet
MAO activity, CSF cytomegalovirus antibody, P-type
(stimulated) atypical lymphocytes, cerebral ventricular
enlargements, abnormal left hemisphere function, impaired
transmission in the corpus callosum, a thickened corpus
callosum, a small cerebellar vermis, decreased cerebral
blood flow and glucose metabolism (by PET scan) in the
frontal lobes, EEG and EP abnormalities (by BEAM), and
pathologically demonstrated fibrillary gliosis in the basal
forebrain, to name a few. Each of these changes are real
in some patients, but their significance is unknown.
However, taken together, they underscore (1) the biological
nature and (2) the heterogeneity of schizophrenia.

BIOCHEMISTRY OF SCHIZOPHRENIA:

The biochemical etiology of schizophrenia is unknown.
Most of the major hypotheses implicate an abnormality of
central neurotransmitters. The current predominant theory
postulates excessive central dopamine (DA) activity (the
Dopamine Hypothesis) and is based on two key findings.

1. The antipsychotic activity of neuroleptic medications
    (eg, phenothiazines) is derived in major part from
    their blockade of postsynaptic dopamine receptors.
2. Amphetamine psychosis often is clinically indistin-
    guishable from an acute paranoid schizophrenic
    psychosis. Amphetamines release central dopamine.
    Also, amphetamines worsen schizophrenia.

Although not conclusive, these results implicate the
dopamine pathways, possibly through (1) a hypersensitivity
of postsynaptic dopamine receptors, (2) an increased number
of receptors, (3) an overactivity of presynaptic dopamine
neurons, or (4) a relative deficiency of dopamine-beta-

hydroxylase (the enzyme which converts DA to NE, forcing DA to become the transmitter in the absense of NE).

Other theories include:

1. Transmethylation hypothesis - Two of the major classes of central transmitters, catecholamines (DA, NE, epinephrine) and indoleamines (serotonin), both produce small amounts of methylated derivatives which are inherently hallucinogenic (eg, mescaline, psilocybin, DMT, bufotenine). Do schizophrenics produce excesses? Are they unable to detoxify those produced? Megavitamin therapy is based on the rationale that certain compounds (eg, nicotinamide) are methyl acceptors and thus, given in large amounts, can "detoxify" the schizophrenic.
2. Excessive central NE (limbic forebrain) occurs in some schizophrenics and decreases with medication and improved clinical state. Thus, NE may be the transmitter to watch, rather than DA.

GENETICS OF SCHIZOPHRENIA:

Schizophrenia has a significant inherited component - probably polygenic.

Consanguinity studies: Schizophrenia is a familial disorder - ie, it "runs in families." The closer the relative, the greater the risk.

Twin studies: Monozygotic twins are 4-6 times more likely to develop illness than dizygotes.

Adoption studies: Children of schizophrenic parents adopted away at birth into normal families have the same increased rate of illness as if they had been raised by their natural parents.

However, a recent debate has questioned the results of all three types of studies (PRO: Karlsson, 1982; Kety, 1983; Grove, 1983; Lowing et al, 1983; Kendler, 1983 - CON: Pope et al, 1982; Abrams and Taylor, 1983; Lidz and Blatt, 1983). Confusion centers on the criteria used to define schizophrenia - the older studies upon which genetic risk factors for schizophrenia are based used criteria other than DSM-III and may have included some patients with affective disorders. Thus, although genetics plays a major role in some patients, the following figures should be considered tentative when applied to all patients.

Genetic Counseling - Lifetime risk of developing schizophrenia:

General population:	1%
Monozygotic twins:	40-50%
Dizygotic twins:	10%
Sibling of a schizophrenic:	10%
Parent of a schizophrenic:	5%
Child of one schizophrenic parent:	10-15%
Child of two schizophrenic parents:	30-40%

Note that 50% of monozygotic twins do not both develop
schizophrenia - thus clearly environment plays a role.
Development of illness reflects nature and nurture.

Although inadequately studied, several non-schizo-
phrenic disorders occur with increased frequency in the
families of schizophrenics and may be related genetically
in some fashion: Schizotypal and Borderline Personality
Disorders (the Schizophrenia Spectrum Disorders); Obsessive
Compulsive Disorder; possibly Antisocial and Paranoid
Personality Disorders.

FAMILY PROCESSES:

Family dynamics and family turbulence play a major
role in producing a relapse or maintaining a remission.
Patients who are discharged to home are more likely to
relapse over the following year than are those who are
placed in a residential setting. Most at risk are patients
from hostile families or families which display excessive
anxiety, overconcern, or overprotectiveness toward the
patient (called expressed emotion or EE - see Leff et al,
1982). Schizophrenic patients frequently do not
"emancipate" from their families.

Some researchers have identified peculiar and pathological styles of communication in these families -
typically, communications are vague and subtly illogical.
Bateson (1956) describes a characteristic "double bind" in
which the patient is frequently required by a key family
member to respond to an overt message which contradicts a
covert message. The significance of this unpleasant bind
in either maintaining or causing (as Bateson suggests) a
Schizophrenic Disorder is unclear. Recent work suggests
that these family communication patterns may be the effect
of having a schizophrenic child, not the cause of it.

DIFFERENTIAL DIAGNOSIS:

Schizophrenia must be differentiated from all of those

conditions which produce active psychoses (see above). Of all the possibilities, be particularly careful to eliminate Schizoaffective Disorder, the Major Affective Disorders, and several organic conditions which may closely mimic schizophrenia - eg, early Huntington's chorea, early Wilson's disease, temporal lobe epilepsy, frontal or temporal lobe tumors, early MS, early SLE, porphyria, general paresis, chronic drug use, chronic alcoholic hallucinosis, and the adult form of metachromatic leukodystrophy. Carefully evaluate catatonia for medical/neurological conditions.

TREATMENT:

Biological methods (see chapter 23): Treat acute psychoses with antipsychotics (equivalent dose range = chlorpromazine 300-1200 mg/day, or more). Relapsing schizophrenics should be considered for antipsychotic drug maintenance - long-acting depot fluphenazine may be the medication of choice. Medication is primarily useful in controlling the "active" symptoms (eg, hallucinations, emotional lability, delusions, etc) and not the "passive" symptoms (eg, anhedonia, social withdrawal) so don't expect too much long-term benefit from meds (except in preventing relapse). Be aware that a chronically excessive dose may chronically hinder patient functioning. A subgroup of schizophrenics may benefit from lithium.

ECT may be useful for rapid control of a few acute psychotics. A very few chronic schizophrenics who respond poorly to medication may improve with ECT - unpredictable.

Psychosocial methods: The essential mode of treatment of schizophrenia is pharmacological. Long-term insight psychotherapy seems to leave the underlying (biological) process unchanged, although it continues to be used (see McGlashan, 1983). Certain other supportive, reality-oriented psychosocial methods are particularly useful adjuncts (May, 1968).

The acutely psychotic patient should be approached cautiously but he should be approached. Keep a comfortable distance from the patient if he appears disturbed by your presence. It is vitally important to establish some communication with these patients.

1. Talk to the patient. Be relaxed, interested, and
   supportive. Give the impression that you believe the
   patient can respond appropriately to you.
2. Be specific. Ask pointed, factual questions. Try to
   identify the patient's major current fears and

concerns but don't be led into a lengthy discussion of complex delusions and hallucinations.
3. Take your time during the interview. Don't rush the patient to respond to each question but do maintain some control over the direction of the conversation.
4. Make some specific observations of the patient's behavior (eg, "you look frightened; you look angry") but don't become involved in lengthy "interpretations." Don't draw incorrect conclusions about the patient's emotional state from inappropriate affect.
5. Explain to the patient what is being done to him, and why.
6. If the conversation is going nowhere (eg, the patient refuses to talk), break off the interview with a positive expectation - eg, "I'll be back to see you in a little while when you are feeling better and able to talk."

If the acutely psychotic patient is delirious, suicidal, homicidal, and/or has no community support - hospitalize. It is usually better to avoid long-term hospitalization if alternate outpatient arrangements are possible: the deleterious effects of chronic hospitalization are real (regression, marked withdrawal, loss of skills, etc), The recent trend has been towards short hospital stays during acute episodes with maintenance as outpatients in between.

When hospitalized, allow the patient as much independence as his behavior permits within the limits of a safe environment. Therapeutic milieus (eg, therapeutic community, token economy, etc) all depend upon community support (staff and patients) - be aware of the patient's behavior and provide helpful "corrective feedback" to him. The milieu is a place for the patient to develop skills in maintaining interpersonal relationships and to learn new methods of coping. The general effectiveness of therapeutic milieus is in doubt although they may be specifically useful for a few patients. Behavior modification has been found clearly effective with some regressed, poorly functioning inpatients at eliminating specific unacceptable behaviors and in teaching low-level personal skills.

Most schizophrenics can be treated as outpatients. Several principles should be kept in mind.

- See the patient frequently enough to safely monitor medication and detect early deterioration (eg, weekly, monthly, or even every several months - dependent upon the patient's course and reliability).

- Communicate with the patient clearly and unambiguously. Be factual and goal-oriented. Avoid extensive discussion of hallucinations and delusions. Help the patient with reality issues - eg, living arrangements, work. Help the patient avoid excessive stress. Recognize that the more productive and skillful the patient, the more likely he is to maintain a recovery - encourage the patient to hold an appropriate job. Provide social skills training.

- Talk about medication - eg, the need for it; the patient's feelings about taking it; etc.

- Develop a consistent, trusting relationship (often difficult). Be empathic over time, even when the patient is being "unreasonable" but also maintain a "professional distance." Be a constant presence.

- Learn the patient's strengths and weaknesses. Teach him to identify an impending decompensation. What are the precipitants, if any? If the patient misses appointments, investigate (he may be relapsing). If the patient is decompensating, be ready to insist on hospitalization. Recognize that over-stimulation and over-independence can precipitate a decompensation. Recognize that these patients are at risk for suicide at times during their illnesses (particularly if they have self-destructive command hallucinations).

- Always evaluate the family. Have they contributed to the patient's decompensation? Can the members deal appropriately with the patient's illness? Are they hostile? Suspicious? Overprotective? Consider family therapy. Family members often need considerable support and understanding themselves. When worked with well, they can be a (the?) major help to the patient (Leff et al, 1982).

- Consider group therapy. The usual orientation is toward support and reality testing. It helps with resocialization, forces interpersonal interaction, and provides support. Several studies have shown it to be effective (in combination with medication) in preventing relapse in outpatients.

- Know and use community resources. Be alert to the devastating effect on the patient of a poor quality of life (eg, does he live in a "psychiatric ghetto?")

- Do not expect too much. Many patients have chronic symptoms.

SCHIZOPHRENIFORM DISORDER

(DSM-III p 199, 295.40)

This disorder is clinically indistinguishable from Schizophrenia and Brief Reactive Psychosis except that the symptoms last more than 2 weeks but less than 6 months. Research (eg, Rosenthal et al, 1968) suggests that this population of patients differs from schizophrenics in several important ways:

1. Symptoms begin and end more abruptly.
2. Symptoms are usually more turbulent and "acute."
3. There is good premorbid adjustment and higher functioning after recovery.
4. There is only a slightly increased prevalence of Schizophrenia in the family. There may be a higher prevalence of affective disorder.

Thus, Schizophreniform Disorder appears to be a separate disease from Schizophrenia. Recognize, however, that many schizophrenic patients pass through a period (ie, the first 6 months) when their diagnosis needs to be Schizophreniform Disorder. Don't miss an organic psychosis.

Treatment is similar to that of an acute schizophrenic episode but the prognosis is better.

BRIEF REACTIVE PSYCHOSIS

(DSM-III p 200, 298.80)

This condition describes those patients who experience an acute psychotic episode lasting less than 2 weeks which immediately follows an important life stress. The illness comes as a surprise - there is usually no suggestion before the stress that the person is likely to "break down," although this disorder is more common in people with a preexisting personality disorder (particularly Histrionic and Borderline types).

The psychosis is typically very turbulent and dramatic with marked emotional lability, bizarre behavior, confused and incoherent speech, transient disorientation and memory loss, and/or brief but striking hallucinations and delusions. Thus, it mimics the acute psychotic onset of a Major Affective Disorder, Schizophreniform Disorder, or Atypical Psychosis and the diagnosis must be changed to one of these if the illness extends beyond 2 weeks. Always carefully rule out OBS and, particularly, drug-related problems.

Treat the acutely psychotic patient with understanding, a secure environment, and antipsychotic medication, if needed. The patient usually recovers completely in several days and the long-term prognosis is good although the patient may be at risk for future brief episodes when equivalently stressed.

SCHIZOAFFECTIVE DISORDER

(DSM-III p 202, 295.70)

This is a vague and poorly defined disorder meant for patients who have evidence of both Schizophrenia and Major Affective Disorder. There are no specific diagnostic criteria - the diagnosis is made by exclusion. These patients may present with an affective disturbance which grades into a purely schizophrenic picture or may display symptoms of both conditions simultaneously. It is a genetically heterogeneous disorder - both schizophrenia and mood disorders occur with increased frequency in family members (Tsuang, 1979). Much work remains to be done to better define this population (Berg et al, 1983).

Treat as one would the equivalent schizophrenic or affective patient. Antipsychotics are generally more useful but lithium has benefited some patients. These patients seem to have a better prognosis than schizophrenics but a poorer outcome than Manic-Depressives.

PARANOID DISORDERS

These patients do not display the pervasive disturbances of mood and thought found in other psychotic conditions. They do not have flat or inappropriate affect, prominent hallucinations, or markedly bizarre delusions. They do have one or more delusions of persecution or infidelity which are:

1. Usually specific - eg, involve a certain person or group, a given place or time, or a particular activity.
2. Usually well organized - eg, the "culprits" have elaborate reasons for what they are doing, which the patient can detail.
3. Usually grandiose - eg, a powerful group is interested just in him.
4. Not bizarre enough to suggest Schizophrenia.

These patients (who tend to be in their 30's and 40's) may be unrecognizable until their delusional system is pointed out by family or friends. Even then the diagnosis may be difficult because they may be too mistrustful to confide in the examiner and don't voluntarily seek treatment. They are frequently hypersensitive, argumentative, and litigious and come to attention through ill-founded legal activities. Although they may perform well occupationally and in areas distant from their delusions, they tend to be social isolates either by preference or as a result of their interpersonal inhospitality (eg, spouses frequently abandon them).

CLASSIFICATION:

PARANOIA (DSM-III p 197, 297.10): Fixed delusions which develop insidiously and last at least 6 months (usually last years).

SHARED PARANOID DISORDER (Folie a deux) (DSM-III p 197, 297.30): The patient adopts the delusional system of another person (usually a dominant spouse).

ACUTE PARANOID DISORDER (DSM-III p 197, 298.30): The paranoid delusional system lasts less than 6 months and usually follows a major life stress.

These conditions appear to form a clinical continuum with conditions like Paranoid Personality Disorder and Paranoid Schizophrenia and delineation of the limits of each syndrome awaits further research (Kendler, 1982). Rule out an affective disorder - morbid jealousy and other paranoid ideas are common in depression. Paranoia is common among the elderly (see chapter 24) and among stimulant drug abusers (Sato et al, 1983). Acute paranoid reactions frequently are seen in patients with mild delirium and in patients who are bedridden (and sensory-deprived).

Etiology is unknown. No genetic or biological factors have been identified. There is a higher incidence among refugee and minority groups and among those with impaired hearing. There is a tendency for their family relationships to be characterized by turbulence, callousness, and coldness yet the significance of this pattern is unclear. Typical defense mechanisms seen in these patients include denial, projection, and regression.

TREATMENT:

Treatment of the paranoid disorders is notoriously difficult. Individual psychotherapy is useful. Emphasis should be on developing a trusting relationship, with the patient seeing the therapist as neutral and accepting. Interfere with the patient's freedom of choice as little as possible. Gradually help the patient see his world from your perspective. These patients are very sensitive to criticism (overt or implied) so this kind of a relationship is extremely difficult to develop and maintain.

Antipsychotic medication may help a few - it may at least take the "energy" out of the delusion. Recent use of antidepressants appears promising (Akiskal et al, 1983) - consider it. Separation of the partners with a shared delusion often produces disappearance of the delusions in the healthier member.

ATYPICAL PSYCHOSIS

(DSM-III p 202, 298.90)

If a psychotic patient does not have an affective disorder, OBS, or one of the disorders in this chapter and is not malingering, he has an Atypical Psychosis. The most common use of this classification is for patients for whom there is insufficient information to make a more specific diagnosis.

REFERENCES

1. Abrams R, Taylor MA: The genetics of schizophrenia: a reassessment using modern criteria. Am J Psychiat 140:171, 1983.
2. Akiskal HS, Arana GW, Baldessarini RJ, Barreira PJ: A clinical report of thymoleptic-responsive atypical paranoid psychosis. Am J Psychiat 140:1187, 1983.
3. Andreasen NC, Olsen S: Negative v positive schizophrenia. Arch Gen Psychiat 39:789, 1982.
4. Arieti S: Interpretation of Schizophrenia, 2nd ed. New York, Basic Books, 1974.
5. Bateson G, Jackson DD, Haley J, Weakland JH: Towards a theory of schizophrenia. Behav Sci 1:251, 1956.
6. Berg E, Lindelium R, Petterson U, Salum I: Schizoaffective psychosis. Acta Psychiatr Scand 67:389, 1983.
7. Bleuler M: The Schizophrenic Disorders. New Haven, Yale Univ Pr, 1978.
8. Gift TE, Strauss JS, Kokes RF, Harder DW, Ritzler BA: Schizophrenia: affect and outcome. Am J Psychiat 137:580, 1980.

9. Grove WM: Comment on Lidz and associates critique of the Danish-American studies of the offspring of schizophrenic parents. Am J Psychiat 140:998, 1983.
10. Henn FA, Nasrallah HA: Schizophrenia as a Brain Disease. New York, Oxford Univ Pr, 1982.
11. Herz MI, Melville C: Relapse in schizophrenia. Am J Psychiat 137:801, 1980.
12. Karlsson JL: Family transmission of schizophrenia: a review and synthesis. Brit J Psychiat 140:600, 1982.
13. Kendler KS: Overview: a current perspective on twin studies of schizophrenia. Am J Psychiat 140:1413, 1983.
14. Kendler KS: Demography of paranoid psychosis (delusional disorder). Arch Gen Psychiat 39:890, 1982.
15. Kendler KS, Gruenberg AM, Strauss JS: An independent analysis of the Copenhagen sample of the Danish adoption study of schizophrenia: V. The relationship between childhood social withdrawal and adult schizophrenia. Arch Gen Psychiat 39:1257, 1982.
16. Kety SS: Mental illness in the biological and adoptive relatives of schizophrenic adoptees: findings relevant to genetic and environmental factors in etiology. Am J Psychiat 140:720, 1983.
17. Leff J, Kuipers L, Berkowitz R, Eberlein-Vries R, Sturgeon D: A controlled trial of social intervention in the families of schizophrenic patients. Brit J Psychiat 141:121, 1982.
18. Lewine R, Burbach D, Meltzer HY: Effect of diagnostic criteria on the ratio of male to female schizophrenic patients. Am J Psychiat 141:84, 1984.
19. Lidz T, Blatt S: Critique of the Danish-American studies of the biological and adoptive relatives of adoptees who became schizophrenic. Am J Psychiat 140:426, 1983.
20. Lowing PA, Mirsky AF, Pereira R: The inheritance of schizophrenia spectrum disorders: a reanalysis of the Danish adoptee study data. Am J Psychiat 140:1167, 1983.
21. Mandel MR, Severe JB, Schooler NR, Gelenberg AJ, Mieske M: Development and prediction of postpsychotic depression in neuroleptic-treated schizophrenics. Arch Gen psychiat 39:197, 1982.
22. May PR: Treatment of Schizophrenia. New York, Science House, 1968.
23. McGlashan TH: Intensive individual psychotherapy of schizophrenia. Arch Gen Psychiat. 40:909, 1983.
24. Parnas J, Schulsinger F, Schulsinger H, Mednick SA, Teasdale TW: Behavioral precursors of schizophrenia spectrum. Arch Gen Psychiat 39:658, 1982.

25. Pope HG, Jonas JM, Cohen BM, Lipinski JF: Failure to find evidence of schizophrenia in first-degree relatives of schizophrenic probands. Am J Psychiat 139:826, 1982.
26. Rosenthal D, Kety SS: The Transmission of Schizophrenia. Oxford, Pergamon Pr, 1968.
27. Sato M, Chen C, Akiyama K, Otsuki S: Acute exacerbation of paranoid psychotic state after long-term abstinence in patients with previous methamphetamine psychosis. Biol Psychiat 18:429, 1983.
28. Seeman MV, McGee H: Treating depression in schizophrenic patients. Am J Psychotherapy 36:14, 1982.
29. Tsuang MT: Schizoaffective disorder. Arch Gen Psychiat 36:633, 1979.
30. Van Kammen DP, Alexander PE, Bunney WE: Lithium treatment in post-psychotic depression. Brit J Psychiat 136:479, 1980.
31. Van Putten T, May PRA: `Akinetic Depression' in schizophrenia. Arch Gen Psychiat 35:1101, 1978.

Chapter 4

Mood Disorders

Patients with disorders of mood are common (10% of the population at any one time) and seen by all medical specialists. It is essential to identify them and either treat or refer appropriately.

Two primary abnormalities of mood are recognized: depression and mania. Both occur on a continuum from normal to the clearly pathological - symptoms in a few patients reach psychotic proportions. Although some patients seem to suffer an extension of normal sadness or elation, discrete syndromes (affective disorders) exist which appear to differ qualitatively and quantitatively from normal processes and require different therapies. A third group consists of those mood disorders which follow medical or other psychiatric processes (secondary disorders).

CLASSIFICATION

Classification of affective disorders is currently unsatisfactory. The two most useful (but overlapping) schemes involve primary-secondary and bipolar-unipolar (used in DSM-III) dichotomies.

PRIMARY-SECONDARY:

Primary Affective Disorder - antedates any non-affective psychiatric or serious medical disorder.

Secondary Affective Disorder - requires preexisting medical or psychiatric illness.

(In practice the chronology, and thus the differentiation, may be uncertain.)

BIPOLAR-UNIPOLAR: (DSM-III)

MAJOR AFFECTIVE DISORDER - <u>major</u> depressive and/or manic signs and symptoms.

<u>Bipolar Disorder</u> (Manic-Depression) - presence or history of mania with or without presence or history of depression.

<u>Unipolar Disorder</u> (Major Depression) - depression alone.

OTHER SPECIFIC AFFECTIVE DISORDER - <u>minor</u> depressive and/or manic signs and symptoms.

<u>Dysthymic Disorder</u> - depression alone.

<u>Cyclothymic Disorder</u> - depressive <u>and</u> hypomanic symptoms in past or present.

ATYPICAL AFFECTIVE DISORDER

ADJUSTMENT DISORDER WITH DEPRESSED MOOD

Major Affective Disorders are primary and often reach psychotic severity. The other disorders are a mix of primary and secondary and are non-psychotic. The DSM-III classification also requires the examiner to specify whether the current bipolar episode is manic, depressed, or mixed; whether the unipolar disorder is a single episode or recurrent; whether either disorder shows psychotic features; and whether a depressive episode meets the criteria for <u>melancholia</u> (profound vegetative and cognitive symptoms including psychomotor retardation or agitation, sleep disturbance, anorexia or weight loss, and/or excessive guilt - see DSM-III p 215). These characteristics are felt to be important in determining treatment and prognosis.

CLINICAL PRESENTATION OF MOOD DISORDERS

There is a core of clinical features common to affective disturbances. Depression can vary from sadness to profound psychotic retardation. Mania can be mild (<u>hypomania</u>) or extend to a manic delirium. However, the Major Affective Disorders have the greater number and severity of symptoms and signs. The most common symptoms and signs of mood disorders include:

Symptoms of depression:

Emotional features
    depressed mood, "blue"
    irritability, anxiety
    anhedonia, loss of interest
    loss of zest
    diminished emotional bonds
    interpersonal withdrawal
    preoccupation with death

Congnitive features
    self-criticism, sense of worthlessness, guilt
    pessimism, hopelessness, despair
    distractible, poor concentration
    uncertain and indecisive
    variable obsessions
    hypochondriacal preoccupations
    memory impairment
    delusions and hallucinations

Vegetative features
    fatigability, no energy
    insomnia or hypersomnia
    anorexia or hyperrexia
    weight loss or gain
    psychomotor retardation
    psychomotor agitation
    impaired libido
    frequent diurnal variation

Signs of depression:

    stooped and slow moving
    tearful, sad facies
    dry mouth and skin
    constipation

Symptoms of mania:

Emotional features
    excited, elevated mood, euphoria
    emotional lability
    rapid, temporary shifts to acute depression
    irritability, low frustration tolerance
    demanding, egocentric

Cognitive features
   elevated self-esteem, grandiosity
   speech disturbances
      loud, word rhyming (clanging)
      pressure of speech
      flight of ideas
      progression to incoherence
   poor judgement, disorganization
   paranoia
   delusions and hallucinations

Physiological features
   boundless energy
   insomnia, little need for sleep
   decreased appetite

Signs of mania:

   psychomotor agitation

A combination of these symptoms often clinches the diagnosis. However, particularly when the symptoms are mild, disorders of mood are frequently missed.

Although many depressed patients complain of depression, some do not and other problems may obscure the diagnosis. Some patients present with alcohol or drug abuse or acting-out behavior. Others, particularly early on, present primarily with anxiety or agitation. Still others, instead of feeling sad, complain of fatigue, insomnia, dyspnea, tachycardia, and vague and/or chronic pains (usually GI, cardiac, headaches, or backaches - all unrelieved by analgesics). People with such presentations (known as masked depressions) often have a personal or family history of depression and frequently respond to antidepressants. Thus, suspect depression in the unimproved patient who has atypical medical symptoms.

Patients with mania rarely complain of their symptoms. They feel too good and are the last people to notice that their behavior is outrageous.

Patient self-rating tests can help determine the severity of a depression: eg, the Beck Depression Inventory (21 questions) and the Zung Self-Rating Depression Scale.

NORMAL AFFECTIVE PROCESSES

Sadness or simple unhappiness affect us all from time to time. The cause is often obvious, the reaction understandable, and improvement follows the disappearance of the cause. However, prolonged unhappiness in response to a chronic stress may be indistinguishable from a minor affective disorder and require treatment. Support and altered life circumstances are the keys to recovery.

Grief or UNCOMPLICATED BEREAVEMENT (DSM-III p 333, V62.82) is a more profound sense of dysphoria which follows a greater loss or trauma and which may produce a full depressive syndrome but, as time distances the precipitating event, the symptoms disappear. This process often takes weeks or months and requires a "working through" which includes disbelief, intense mourning, and eventual resolution (see chapter 10). If the grieving process is interrupted, the period of grief may be prolonged or may develop into a major depressive disorder.

There is no generally accepted equivalent non-pathological manic process although some people do react to stress with overactivity.

MINOR AFFECTIVE DISORDERS

DEPRESSION:

The common chronic non-psychotic disorder of lowered mood and/or anhedonia is DYSTHYMIC DISORDER (Depressive Neurosis) (DSM-III p 220, 300.40). These patients feel depressed, have difficulty falling asleep, characteristically feel best in the morning and despondent in the afternoon and evening, and can display any of the non-psychotic symptoms and signs of depression. Symptoms must have been present, at least intermittently, for two or more years. It is more common in women (3-4:1), often develops for the first time in the late 20's or 30's, and begins insidiously, frequently in a person predisposed to depression by:

- major loss in childhood; eg, parent.
- recent loss; eg, health, job, spouse.
- chronic stress; eg, medical disorder.
- psychiatric susceptibility; eg, personality disorders of histrionic, compulsive, and dependent types; alcohol and drug abuse; Major Depression in partial remission; obsessive compulsive disorder. It frequently coexists with these conditions.

It is similar to but less severe than a Major Depression. However, 10-15% of patients who experience major depression will clear incompletely, and chronically suffer a residue of dysthymic disorder ("double depression" - see Keller et al, 1983).

Dysthymic disorder must be differentiated from ADJUSTMENT DISORDER WITH DEPRESSED MOOD (DSM-III p 301, 309.00). This disorder occurs in an adequately functioning individual shortly after a readily identifiable, causative stress, results in impaired functioning, and resolves as the stress disappears. These patients present a depressive syndrome midway between normal sadness and major depression. If social withdrawal predominates without strong feelings of depression, the patient may have ADJUSTMENT DISORDER WITH WITHDRAWAL (DSM-III p 302, 309.83).

MANIA:

CYCLOTHYMIC DISORDER (DSM-III p 218, 301.13) requires the presence of mild depression and hypomania, separately or intermixed, continuously or intermittantly over at least a 2 year period. It usually begins in the 20's in patients (females 2:1) with a family history of major affective disorder and forms a chronically disabling pattern which yields troubled interpersonal relationships, job instability, occasional suicide attempts and short hospitalizations, and a markedly increased risk of drug and alcohol abuse.

MAJOR AFFECTIVE DISORDERS

Patients with major affective disorders are profoundly depressed or excited. Clinical presentations and genetic studies support two distinct groups, MAJOR DEPRESSION (unipolar) (DSM-III p 218, 296.2 and 296.3) and BIPOLAR DISORDER (DSM-III p 217, 296.4-6), yet some question this dichotomy. The lifetime risk in the general population for a major depression may be as high as 20% for females and 10% for males - ten times more frequent than bipolar disorder. 15% of the patients kill themselves.

MAJOR DEPRESSION:

These patients have many of the more serious depressive symptoms and signs yet their clinical presentations can vary markedly - from profound retardation and withdrawal to irritable, unrelieved agitation. A presumed precipitating event occurs in 25% (50% among the elderly). A diurnal variation is common, with the most severe symptoms early in the day. Some fail to recognize their depression, complaining instead of their "insides rotting out" or their "minds going crazy," yet the profound affective disturbance is usually recognizable to the observer. A thought disorder is often, but not invariably, present and delusions are usually affect-laden and mood congruent. Hallucinations are uncommon, auditory, and usually have a self-condemning or paranoid content. Depressed elderly may present primarily with retardation, memory impairment, and mild disorientation (pseudodementia).

The disorder can occur at any age with the majority of cases spread evenly throughout the adult years and with females affected 2:1. Unlike schizophrenia, it occurs more frequently in the higher social strata. Family and twin studies strongly suggest a genetic factor - increased incidence of major depression, alcoholism, and possibly antisocial personality disorder in relatives (the "depressive spectrum" disorders). The prevalence of affective illness in first-degree relatives is 13% contrasted with 1% in the general population. Alcoholism and chronic stress predispose to the development of the illness.

Fewer than 40% of patients will have only one episode (M.D., SINGLE EPISODE, 296.2) with the rest having two or more attacks (M.D., RECURRENT, 296.3). Most patients clear between episodes, some remain mildly depressed (10-15%), and a few are chronically, severely depressed. Most attacks begin gradually over 1-3 weeks and, untreated, last from 3-8 months, or longer. These patients are often incapacitated during an episode and are at great risk of suicide.

Postpartum depression is a severe depression beginning 1-2 weeks after delivery, usually of the second or third child. Affected women are at risk for repeat episodes with future births.

The apparent biological nature of many serious depressions is reflected in the recent development of several putative biological tests for depression: the dexamethasone suppression test (DST - positive test is the failure of normal suppression of plasma cortisol 6-24 hours after an oral dose of dexamethasone); urinary MHPG (3-methoxy-4-hydroxyphenyleneglycol - a catabolite of norepinephrine felt to be low in some depressions); urinary phenyl acetate (PAA - low in some depressions; see Sabelli et al, 1983); TRH test (blunted TSH and GH responses to exogenous TRH suggest unipolar depression; see Gold et al, 1981); blunted ITT (glucose response to IV insulin tolerance test is reduced in some depressions; see Lewis et al, 1983); REM latency (time to initiation of REM sleep is decreased in some depressions; see Kupfer et al, 1982); and

amphetamine test (some depressed patients briefly improve
when given 10 mg of amphetamine). Unfortunately, these
tests have little routine clinical utility. They all
suffer from inadequate sensitivity and specificity (too
many false positives and negatives). However, each further
emphasizes that biology plays a role in many depressions.
Moreover, a combination of tests (eg; DST, PAA, and MHPG)
may help clarify issues in the occasional diagnostically
complex or treatment resistant patient.

BIPOLAR DISORDER:

     Mania, at some time severe enough to produce compro-
mised functioning, is necessary for this diagnosis, but
80-90% of patients also have periods of depression (B.D.,
DEPRESSED, 296.5). Early on the mania resembles normal
euphoria but gradually it becomes uncontrolled and psychotic
(B.D., MANIC, 296.4). 20% of manics have hallucinations
and/or delusions. A severe mania may be indistinguishable
from an organic delirium - ie, acute delirious mania
(sudden onset, anorexia, insomnia, disorientation,
paranoia, hallucinations and delusions). The depression is
usually profound but may present as a mild depressive
syndrome. The attacks are usually separated by months or
years but the patient occasionally may cycle from one to
the other over days or actually present contrasting
symptoms simultaneously (eg, spirited singing intermixed
with crying) (B.D., MIXED, 296.6). Pure manic syndromes
(patients who have had only mania - unipolar mania) occur
clinically but are probably not a separate entity.

     The lifetime risk for developing bipolar disorder is
approximately 1%. The importance of genetic factors is
well documented. First-degree relatives are at risk for
bipolar disorder, major depression, cyclothymic disorder,
and alcoholism with a general prevalence of affective
illness of 20%. In contrast with major depression,
male:female is 1:1. The type of inheritance is uncertain -
probably polygenic although there is controversial data
suggesting an X-linked dominance with incomplete
penetrance, linked to color blindness and Xg blood group.

     The first episode is usually before age 30, is often
manic, begins quickly, and resolves in 2-4 months if untreated. Most patients go on to have a majority of
depressive episodes. Suicide is the major risk during
periods of depression. Legal difficulties and drug and
alcohol abuse (as well as suicide) occur with manic periods.

ATYPICAL AFFECTIVE DISORDER

ATYPICAL BIPOLAR DISORDER (DSM-III p 223, 296.70) and ATYPICAL DEPRESSION (DSM-III p 223, 296.82) include the remaining affective presentations.

DIFFERENTIAL DIAGNOSIS

DEPRESSION:

Psychiatric Syndromes:

Schizophrenic Disorders - particularly catatonics, but any type can look or be depressed during or after an episode. Poor premorbid adjustment, formal thought disorder with well-formed delusions and complex hallucinations, lack of cyclic history, and no family history for affective disorder all suggest schizophrenia.

Schizoaffective Disorder - a psychotic disorder that does not meet the criteria for an affective or schizophrenic disorder but which contains features of both.

Generalized Anxiety Disorder - anxiety appears first and predominates. With the anxious patient, always consider depression.

Alcoholism - alcoholism and depression are both often present.

Obsessive Compulsive Neurosis; Histrionic and Compulsive Personality Disorders - are the full syndromes present?

Dementia - "pseudodepression" is common and differentiation is tricky, particularly in the elderly. Check for memory impairment and disorientation.

Physical Syndromes (Organic Affective Syndromes):

Tumors - particularly of brain and lung, carcinoma of pancreas.

Infections - influenza, syphilis, pneumonia, encephalitis, mononucleosis, hepatitis.

Medication - oral contraceptives, corticosteroids, reserpine (6% of patients), alphamethyldopa, guanethidine, levodopa, indomethacin, opiates, benzodiazepines, propranolol, anticholinesterases, amphetamine withdrawal.

Endocrine disorders - Cushing's disease or exogenous steroids, hypothyroidism, slow form of hyperthyroidism, hyperparathyroidism (symptoms parallel levels of serum calcium), diabetes, Turner's syndrome.

Blood - anemia (particularly Pernicious Anemia).
Nutrition and electrolytes - pellagra, hyponatremia,
   hypokalemia, hypercalcemia, inappropriate ADH.
Misc. - MS, heavy metal poisoning, Parkinson's disease,
   cerebrovascular disease.

MANIA:

Psychiatric Syndromes:

Schizophrenic Disorders - often indistinguishable in
   acute cases. Check past personal and family history.
Schizoaffective Disorder

Organic Affective Syndromes:

Tumors - of brain.
Infections - encephalitis, syphilis (20% of patients
   with general paresis).
Medication - steroids, amphetamines, hallucinogens,
   various toxic deliriums.
Misc. - MS, Wilson's disease, hyperthyroidism,
   psychomotor epilepsy, head trauma.

PSYCHOBIOLOGICAL THEORIES

Psychoanalytic theory (Freud) postulates that a
depressed patient has suffered a real or imagined loss of
an ambivalently loved object, has reacted with unconscious
rage which was then turned against the self, and this has
resulted in a lowered self-esteem and depression.
Cognitive theory (A. Beck) postulates a "cognitive triad"
of distorted perceptions in which (1) a person's negative
interpretation of his own life experiences causes (2) a
devaluation of himself which causes (3) depression.

Promising but unproven biological theories focus on
brain norepinephrine (NE) and serotonin (5-HT) abnormalities.
Biological and psychological theories need not be mutually
exclusive. The catecholamine hypothesis (J. Schildkraut,
1965) suggests that low brain NE levels cause depression
and elevated levels cause mania, however, urinary MHPG
levels (a major metabolite of NE) are low in only some
depressions. The indoleamine hypothesis holds that low
cerebral 5-HT (or the primary metabolite, 5-HIAA) causes
depression and elevation causes mania, yet exceptions
occur. The permissive hypothesis postulates that lowered
NE produces depression and raised NE causes mania only if
5-HT levels are low. The known mechanisms of action of
antidepressants support these theories - tricyclics block

NE and 5-HT reuptake and MAOIs block oxidation of NE.
Also, two biologically distinct subtypes of depression may
exist - one with low CFS 5-HIAA (and responding to the
relatively serotonin specific antidepressant,
amitriptyline) and one with low urinary MHPG (and
responding to the NE blocking antidepressant, desipramine),
although those findings are disputed.

TREATMENT OF DEPRESSION

Evaluate medically and psychiatrically to rule out
secondary depression and to attempt to identify an
affective syndrome. Always ask about vegetative features
and evaluate suicidal potential (see chapter 7). If the
patient is (1) incapacitated by the disorder, (2) has a
destructive home environment or limited environmental
support, (3) is a suicide risk, or (4) has an associated
medical illness requiring treatment - hospitalize. All
depressed patients should receive psychotherapy - some must
receive physical therapies in addition. The specific
modalities used to treat depend on the diagnosis, severity,
patient's age, and past responses to therapy.

PSYCHOLOGICAL THERAPIES:

Supportive psychotherapy is always indicated. Be
warm, empathic, understanding, and optimistic. Help the
patient to identify and express concerns and to ventilate.
Identify precipitating factors and help correct. Help
solve external problems (eg, rent, job) - be directive,
particularly during the acute episode and if the patient is
immobilized. Train the patient to recognize signs of
future decompensation. See the patient frequently (1-3X/wk
initially) and regularly but not interminably - be
available. Recognize that some depressed patients can
provoke anger in you (via anger, hostility, unreasonable
demands, etc) - watch for it. Long-term insight-oriented
psychotherapy may be of value in selected chronic minor
depressions and some conflicted patients with a major
depression in remission.

Behavior therapy may help mild to moderately severe
depressives. Felt to be "learned helplessness,"
depressions are treated by giving patients skill training
and providing success experiences. Cognitive therapy is
clearly effective with many patients. The patient is
trained to recognize and eliminate negative expectations.

Recent studies suggest that partial sleep deprivation
(awaken midway through the night and keep up until the next

evening) helps lessen the symptoms of a major depression
(Schilgen and Tolle, 1980). Physical exercise (running,
swimming) may produce improvement in depression for poorly
understood biological reasons.

PHYSICAL THERAPIES:

All major and most chronic or unimproved minor
depressions require a trial of antidepressants (70-80% of
patients respond), even though an apparent precipitant of
the depression is identified. Two types are available:
tricyclic antidepressants and monoamine oxidase inhibitors
(see chapter 23). Begin with a tricyclic antidepressant
but consider a trial with a different tricyclic or an MAOI
(particularly in "atypical" depressions) if the first drug
fails. Antidepressant medication may precipitate a manic
episode in bipolar patients. Maintain for several months
after remission (longer in chronic cases) at half the acute
dose, then taper slowly. T3, coupled with an antidepressant, can induce a remission in an otherwise refractory
patient (Goodwin et al, 1982).

Lithium (see chapter 23) is moderately effective at
maintaining remission in bipolar and some unipolar
patients. Antidepressants and lithium may be started
concurrently, and the lithium continued after remission.
Lithium may be useful in treating acute bipolar depressions
and a few unipolar depressions, but it may exacerbate
symptoms in some patients. Psychotic, paranoid, or very
agitated patients may require an antipsychotic, alone or
with an antidepressant, lithium, or ECT - an antidepressant
alone is usually not sufficient.

Electroconvulsive therapy (ECT) (see chapter 23) may
be the treatment of choice (1) if medication fails after a
3-4 week trial, (2) if the patient's condition demands an
immediate remission (eg, acutely suicidal), (3) in some
psychotic depressions, or (4) in patients who can't
tolerate medication (eg, some elderly cardiac patients).
60-75% of these patients respond.

TREATMENT OF MANIA

Evaluate carefully but quickly. Is the patient
medically ill or taking drugs? Has he been manic before?
Is he taking lithium? What is the blood level?

If hypomanic, consider outpatient treatment. Send
home with family. Sedate with antipsychotic medication;
eg, haloperidol 3-20 mg daily. Begin lithium carbonate.

If manic, hospitalize.   Is patient debilitated?
Seriously sleep deprived?

1. Medicate acutely with antipsychotics (large doses
   often required; eg, haloperidol 10-40 mg or more,
   during first 24 hrs).
2. Be relaxed, reasonable, and controlled. Treat in
   quiet setting with minimal stimuli. Set firm
   limits.
3. Begin lithium carbonate; however, as many as 30% of
   manics stay partially symptomatic in spite of
   lithium.

REFERENCES

1. Aggernaes H, et al: Dexamethasone suppression test and
    TRH test in endogenous depression. Acta Psychiatr Scand
    67:258, 1983.
2. Akiskal HS: Dysthymic disorder: psychopathology of
    proposed chronic depressive states. Am J Psychiat
    140:11, 1983.
3. Akiskal HS, Hirschfeld RMA, Yerevanian BI: The
    relationship of personality to affective disorders.
    Arch Gen Psychiat 40:801, 1983.
4. Akiskal HS, Rosenthal RH, Rosenthal TL, et al:
    Differentiation of primary affective illness from
    situational, symptomatic, and secondary depressions.
    Arch Gen Psychiat 36:635, 1979.
5. Arieti S, Bemporad J: Severe and Mild Depression. New
    York, Basic Books, 1978.
6. Beeber AR, Pies RW: The nonmelancholic depressive
    syndromes. J Nerv Ment Dis 171:3, 1983.
7. Bond TC: Recognition of acute delirious mania. Arch Gen
    Psychiat 37:553, 1980.
8. Brown RP, Sweeney J, Loutash E, Kocsis J, Frances A:
    Involutional melancholia revisited. Am J Psychiat
    141:24, 1984.
9. Carroll BJ: The dexamethasone suppression test for
    melancholia. Brit J Psychiat 140:292, 1982.
10. Cassano GB, Maggini C, Akiskal HS: Short-term,
    subchronic, and chronic sequelae of affective
    disorders. Psychiatric Clin N Am 6:55, 1983.
11. Davidson JRT, Miller RD, Turnbull CD, Sullivan JL:
    Atypical depression. Arch Gen Psychiat 39:527, 1982.
12. Dietch JT, Zetin M: Diagnosis of organic depressive
    disorders. Psychosomatics 24:971, 1983.
13. Gold MS, et al: The TRH test in the diagnosis of major
    and minor depression. Psychoneuroendocrinology 6:159,
    1981.

14. Goodwin FK, Prange AJ, Post RM, Muscettola G, Lipton MA: Potentiation of antidepressant effects by L-triiodothyronine in tricyclic nonresponders. Am J Psychiat 139:34, 1982.
15. Greden JF, Gardner R, King D, Grunhaus L, Carroll BJ, Kronfol Z: Dexamethasone suppression tests in antidepressant treatment of melancholia. Arch Gen Psychiat 40:493, 1983.
16. Hirschfeld RMA, Klerman GL, Clayton PJ, Keller MB: Personality and depression. Arch Gen Psychiat 40:993, 1983.
17. Hirschfeld RMA, Cross CK: Epidemiology of affective disorders. Arch Gen Psychiat 39:35, 1982.
18. Keller MB, Lavori PW, Endicott J, Coryell W, Klerman BL: "Double depression": two-year follow-up. Am J Psychiat 140:689, 1983.
19. Koslow SH, Maas JW, Bowden CL, Davis JM, Henin I, Javaid J: CSF and urinary biogenic amines and metabolites in depression and mania. Arch Gen Psychiat 40:999, 1983.
20. Kupfer DJ, Shaw DH, Ulrich R, Coble PA, Spiker DG: Application of automated REM analysis in depression. Arch Gen Psychiat 39:569, 1982.
21. Lewis DA, Kathol RG, Sherman BM, Winokur G, Schlesser MA: Differentiation of depressive subtypes by insulin insensitivity in the recovered phase. Arch Gen Psychiat 40:167, 1983.
22. Nurnberger J, Roose SP, Dunner DL, Fieve RR: Unipolar mania: a distinct clinical entity? Am J Psychiat 136:1420, 1979.
23. Rush AJ: Cognitive therapy of depression: rationale, techniques, and efficacy. Psychiatric Clin N Am 6:105, 1983.
24. Sabelli HC, Fawcett J, Gusovsky F, Javaid J, Edwards J, Jeffriess H: Uninary phenyl acetate: a diagnostic test for depression? Science 220:1187, 1983.
25. Schildkraut JJ: The catecholamine hypothesis of affective disorders: a review of supporting evidence. Am J Psychiat 122:509, 1965.
26. Schilgen B, Tolle R: Partial sleep deprivation as therapy for depression. Arch Gen Psychiat 37:267, 1980.
27. Schmidt MM, Miller WR: Amount of therapist contact and outcome in a multidimensional depression treatment program. Acta Psychiatr Scand 67:319, 1983.
28. Simons AD, Garfield SL, Murphy GE: The process of change in cognitive therapy and pharmacotherapy for depression. Arch Gen Psychiat 41:45, 1984.
29. Weissman MM, et al: Psychiatric disorders in the relatives of probands with affective disorders. Arch Gen Psychiat 41:13, 1984.

Chapter 5

Delirium and Other Organic Brain Syndromes

Organic brain syndromes (OBS) are mental disorders of various types caused by a wide range of organic pathology. The most common types are delirium (see below), dementia (see chapter 6), and intoxication and withdrawal (see chapters 16 and 17).

These syndromes are common, particularly among the elderly (10-15% of all acute medical inpatients develop a degree of OBS - usually delirium). Although some of these conditions have fairly characteristic clinical presentations, it is necessary to identify a putative organic cause before making the diagnosis. Delirium is usually brief and reversible and dementia is longer-lasting and more likely to be irreversible yet none of these characterizations is completely true (eg, 15-20% of dementias are reversible). These conditions are clinically defined and their course and characteristics are dependent upon the nature, severity, course, and location of the causative organic pathology.

DELIRIUM
(DSM-III p 104, 293.00)

This is a very common condition, particularly among persons who are physically ill. These patients may present with confused, bizarre, and "wild" behavior which may lead a physician who is unfamiliar with delirium to conclude that the patient has a serious functional psychiatric illness. Other delirious patients may appear perfectly well or even somnolent during the day, only to decompensate dramatically in the middle of the night. Still other patients may be having increasing difficulty functioning due to a mild delirium which is only revealed by specific mental status testing. Synonyms include acute brain syndrome, toxic psychosis, acute confusional state, and metabolic encephalopathy.

DIAGNOSIS:

Delirium is a rapidly developing disorder of disturbed attention which fluctuates with time. Although the clinical presentation of delirium differs considerably from patient to patient, there are several characteristic features which help make the diagnosis.

- Clouding of consciousness: The patient is not normally alert and may appear bewildered and confused. He may have noticeably decreased alertness (grading into stupor) or he may be hyperalert. Observe the patient.

- Attention deficit: The patient usually is very distractible and unable to focus his attention sufficiently or for a long enough time to follow a train of thought or to understand what is occurring around him. The patient's thinking is thus typically disordered. Have the patient do serial 7's and/or a Random Letter Test.

- Perceptual disturbances: These are common and include misinterpretations of environmental events, illusions (eg, the curtain blows and the patient believes someone is climbing in the window), and hallucinations (usually visual). The patient may or may not recognize these misperceptions as unreal.

- Sleep-wake alteration: Insomnia is almost always present (all symptoms are usually worse at night and in the dark) while marked drowsiness may also occur.

- Disorientation: Most frequently to time but also to place, situation, and (lastly) person. Ask for the date, time, and day of the week. "What place is this?" etc.

- Memory impairment: The patient typically has a recent memory deficit and usually denies it (he may confabulate and may want to talk about the distant past). Ask about the recent past - eg, "Who brought you to the hospital? Did you have any tests yesterday? What did you have for breakfast?" etc. Name four objects and two words and ask the patient for them in 5 minutes. Does he remember your name?

- Incoherence: The patient may attempt to communicate but the speech may be confused or even unintelligible. Verbal perseveration may occur.

- Altered psychomotor activity: Most delirious patients are restless and agitated and may display perseveration of motion; some may be excessively somnolent; and some

may fluctuate from one to the other (usually restless
at night and sleepy during the day).

- <u>Fluctuations</u>: Most of the characteristics listed above
  vary in severity over hours and days.

A delirium usually develops over days and <u>may</u> precede
signs of the organic condition causing it. If a delirium
is recognized, look for the etiology. Usually it lasts
less than a week (depending on the cause). Many of these
patients are significantly anxious or frightened by their
experiences, may become combative, and may develop some
delusional ideas based on their misperceptions. A few
patients become dangerously suicidal - watch for it.
Environmental conditions can significantly alter the
presentation of a delirium. Change of setting (eg, moving
out of familiar surroundings), overstimulation, and
understimulation (eg, darkness, sensory deprivation) can
all worsen the symptoms, as can stress of any kind.

It is necessary to have a high index of suspicion and
to ask specific mental status questions if you are going to
identify delirium early - do so tactfully since many
patients defensively resist this probing. The early,
prodromal symptoms which should alert you to a developing
delirium include (Lipowski, 1980):

    restlessness (particularly at night), anxiety
    daytime somnolence
    insomnia, vivid dreams and nightmares
    hypersensitivity to light and sound
    fleeting illusions and hallucinations
    distractibility; difficulty in thinking clearly

The EEG, although usually not necessary to make the
diagnosis, has a characteristic pattern of diffuse slowing
and can help if there is a question of the presence of a
functional psychosis, drug use, or a dissociative state.
There may also be a tremor, asterixis, diaphoresis,
tachycardia, elevated BP, tachypnea, and flushing.

ETIOLOGY AND DIFFERENTIAL DIAGNOSIS:

The presence of a delirium usually means that the
patient is seriously medically ill. Delirium is a
diagnosis that immediately demands a search for causes.
Most causes produce diffuse cerebral impairment and lie
<u>outside</u> the CNS - usually due to some form of deranged
<u>metabolism</u> (eg, infection, fever, hypoxia, hypoglycemia,
drug withdrawal states, hepatic encephalopathy). The
specific potential etiologies are too numerous to list

(consult a more complete source - eg, Lipowski, Delirium, 1980) although usually the cause is evident. These patients all deserve a thorough physical and laboratory examination.

The major problem in differential diagnosis is in distinguishing a delirium from an acute functional psychosis. The delirious patient is usually more acute and confused and the hallucinations are usually more disorganized and are more likely to be visual. Patients with functional psychoses usually don't have confusion, disorientation, and illusions, and they are more likely to have a formal thought disorder. Always check the personal and family history for serious psychiatric illness.

TREATMENT:

- Provide adequate medical care for an identified cause of the delirium. Patients with delirium have an increased mortality rate (Waddington, 1982).
- Provide for the patient's safety. Maintain around-the-clock observation (particularly at night). This may require someone in the room constantly - preferably someone with whom the patient is familiar. Use restraints only if absolutely necessary (they frequently increase agitation).
- Keep patient in a quiet, well-lighted room. Keep familiar objects around and use the same treatment personnel, if possible.
- Frequently (and tactfully) re-orient the patient. Introduce yourself again and describe what you are doing and why.
- Anticipate the patient's anxiety and reassure him. Be calm and sympathetic.
- Medication should be used cautiously. Use low doses. If psychotic features are prevalent, consider haloperidol or chlorpromazine. If sedation is called for (usually for marked anxiety), consider the benzodiazepines (eg, diazepam or chlordiazepoxide).

The following organic brain syndromes are considerably less common than delirium, dementia, and the substance abuse syndromes of intoxication and withdrawal. They are also more likely to be associated with focal organic pathology and with a few specific medical or neurological diseases.

AMNESTIC SYNDROME

(DSM-III p 112, 294.00)

These patients have severe memory deficits which usually appear suddenly following a CNS insult and which may be chronic. The deficits are <u>both</u> retrograde (old, past memories - ask about childhood, schooling, etc) and anterograde (new memory - ask the patient to remember several facts for 5-10 minutes). The patients are often unaware that their memory is impaired. Unlike delirium, the sensorium is usually clear, although there may be disorientation. Unlike dementia, serious memory loss occurs without intellectual or other associated changes.

There are numerous potential causes which include CNS trauma, hypoxia, herpes simplex encephalitis, and some substance abuse (particularly alcohol and sedative-hypnotic abuse - see chapters 16 and 17). Bilateral lesions of the medial temporal and/or diencephalic regions appear to be required. Treatment consists of correcting any medical/ organic causes and waiting.

ORGANIC HALLUCINOSIS

(DSM-III p 115, 293.82)

The only characteristic symptom is the presence of hallucinations (of any type but usually visual or auditory) although they may be accompanied by concern or anxiety. The patient is usually (but not always) aware of the symptom's unreality. The most common etiology is drug abuse (usually hallucinogens) or sensory deprivation (eg, deafness). It is easily distinguished from delirium and the psychotic disorders by the absence of other related symptoms.

ORGANIC PERSONALITY SYNDROME

(DSM-III p 118, 310.10)

These patients display a personality <u>change</u> or a marked exacerbation of previous personality characteristics. Most commonly this takes the form of a loss of control over impulses and emotions or the development of apathy, irritability, or indifference. Impairment of social judgement is common. The usual cause is frontal lobe damage (the frontal lobe syndrome) due to tumors, CNS trauma, general paresis, normal pressure

hydrocephalus, Huntington's chorea, or MS. Be careful not
to mistake for mild delirium or the early changes of
dementia, schizophrenia, or Major Affective Disorder.

ORGANIC DELUSIONAL SYNDROME

(DSM-III p 114, 293.81)

This syndrome may mimic schizophrenia - the presence
of delusions (usually paranoid) in a clear sensorium is the
predominant symptom but almost any psychotic-like symptom
can occur. The most common cause is amphetamine abuse but
it may also be due to abuse of other drugs (eg, cocaine,
cannabis), encephalitis, psychomotor epilepsy, and
occasionally other CNS pathology. Without good evidence of
organic pathology, it is very difficult to differentiate
this syndrome from a functional psychosis.

ORGANIC AFFECTIVE SYNDROME

(DSM-III p 117, 293.83)

This syndrome typically mimics a depression or mania.
To make the diagnosis, it is necessary to identify a likely
organic factor as causative. Numerous drugs and medical
conditions can cause this syndrome (see chapters 13, 14,
15).

REFERENCES

1. Dubin WR, Weiss KJ, Zeccardi JA: Organic brain
    syndrome: the psychiatric imposter. JAMA 249:60, 1983.
2. Henker FO: Acute brain syndromes. J Clin Psychiat
    54:117, 1979.
3. Jacob JW, Bernhad MR, Delgado A, Strain JJ: Screening
    for organic mental syndromes in the medically ill. Ann
    Internal Med 86:40, 1977.
4. Lipowski ZJ: Delirium. Springfield, Ill, Charles C
    Thomas Pub, 1980.
5. Lipowski ZJ: A new look at organic brain syndromes. Am
    J Psychiat 137:674, 1980.
6. Lipowski ZJ: Transient cognitive disorders (delirium,
    acute confusional states) in the elderly. Am J Psychiat
    140:1426, 1983.
7. Victor M: The amnestic syndrome and its anatomical
    basis. Can Med Assoc J 100:1115, 1969.
8. Weddington WW: The mortality of delirium: an
    underappreciated problem? Psychosomatics 23:1232, 1982.

Chapter 6

Dementia

DEMENTIA (DSM-III p 107, 294.10) results from a broad loss of intellectual functions due to diffuse organic disease of the cerebral hemispheres which is of sufficient severity to impair social and/or occupational functioning. Dementia is a clinical presentation demanding a diagnosis - not a diagnosis itself. Causes are numerous but clinical presentations are remarkably similar. 60% of dementias are irreversible but, since 25% are controllable and 15% are reversible, treatable causes must be identified.

MAKING THE DIAGNOSIS

Dementia usually develops slowly and is easily overlooked. A rapid onset suggests a recent (and possibly treatable) insult although frequently a mild, unrecognized dementia is made worse and obvious by a medical illness (eg, pneumonia, CHF). Always interview the family - they frequently notice changes (in personality, memory, etc) of which the patient is unaware. Unlike Delirium, there is no clouding of consciousness - make sure the patient is alert.

EARLY - Effects include: subtle changes in personality, impaired social skills, a decrease in the range of interests and enthusiasms, lability and shallowness of affect, agitation, numerous somatic complaints, vague psychiatric symptoms, and a gradual loss of intellectual skills and acuity. These are often first noticed in work settings where performance is required. Patients may recognize a loss of abilities initially but vigorously deny it. Early dementia often precipitates a depression (Reifler et al, 1982). Remember: early dementia may present primarily with emotional (usually depressive) rather than cognitive symptoms, but also emotional disorders may mimic early dementia - don't under- or over-diagnose it.

LATE - Parts of the full picture emerge:

Memory loss - Usually immediate and recent memory loss
but gradually involving remote recall (medial temporal
and diencephalic regions involved). Does patient
forget appointments, the news, people he has just met,
or places he has just been? Patient may confabulate,
so check his information.

Ask patient to (1) repeat digits (normal - remember
6 forward, 4 backward) and (2) recall 2 words and 3
objects after 5 minutes. Does he know your name? the
nurse? this place? the names of his visitors? last
night's meal? Does he know his birthdate? his home-
town? the name of his high school?

Changes in mood and personality - Often exaggeration of
previous personality (eg, more compulsive or more
excitable). Depression, anxiety, and/or irritability
early on - later, withdrawal and apathy. Has the
patient become sloppy, belligerent, thoughtless of
others, paranoid, socially inappropriate, fearful?
Does he lack initiative or interest? use vulgar
language or jokes?

Loss of orientation - Particularly time (of day, day of
week, date, season) but also place ("What place is
this?") and, when severe, person. Has he been getting
lost - in new places? in old neighborhood? at home?
Does he know why he is here (situation)? He may not
sleep well, wander around at night, and get lost.

Intellectual impairment - Patient is "less sharp" than he
used to be. Does he have trouble doing things he
could previously do easily? General information (last
5 presidents, 6 large US cities)? Calculations
(multiplication tables, serial 7's, make change)?
Similarities (how are a ball and an orange alike? a
mouse and an elephant? a fly and a tree?).

Compromised judgement - Doesn't anticipate consequences.
Does he act impulsively? "What should you do if you
found a stamped, addressed envelope?; if you noticed a
fire in a theater?"

Psychotic symptoms - Hallucinations (usually simple),
illusions, delusions, unshakable preoccupations, ideas
of reference.

Language impairment - Often vague and imprecise;
occasionally almost mute. Is there perseveration,
blocking, or aphasia?

Ask about history of chronic medical or psychiatric disease, family psychiatric illness, drug or alcohol abuse, head injury, exposure to toxins.

PHYSICAL EXAMINATION:

Examine for the numerous medical causes of dementia - eg, endocrine, heart, kidney, lung, liver, infection (see below). Always perform a careful neurologic exam - identify any focal CNS causes of dementia. Always test for sense of smell (1st cranial nerve) - may identify a large, unrecognized frontal lobe lesion. Always test hearing. Advanced diffuse disease displays ataxia, facial grimaces, agnosias, apraxias, motor impersistence, and/or perseveration, and pathological reflexes (grasp, snout, suck, glabella tap, tonic foot, etc). Recognize that all types of physical illnesses occur more frequently in the demented (reasons for this are unclear). Survival time is reduced.

LABORATORY EXAMINATION:

Select tests based on suspected etiology. Consider screening with (Wells, 1977): ESR, CBC, STS, SMA-12, T3T4, Vitamin B12 and folate assays, UA, chest X-ray, and CT scan. Other tests based on likely causes include drug levels, EEG (20% of all elderly have an abnormal EEG), LP, arteriography, etc. The EEG is useful for identifying pathology in the usually silent CNS areas (frontal and temporal lobes) - investigate further if the dementia is mild but the EEG is grossly abnormal.

PSYCHOLOGICAL TESTING:

These can (1) help identify a focal lesion, (2) provide a baseline, (3) help with the diagnosis, and (4) identify strengths to be used in planning treatment. Useful tests include: WAIS, Bender-Gestalt Test, the Luria test, Halstead and Reitan Batteries (very time consuming). Don't use routinely. A brief but useful screening test is the Mini-Mental State Exam (Folstein et al, 1975). Patients with even mild dementia often will show impaired constructional ability thus have them draw simple figures (eg, a diamond, cross, and cube - can be done on initial interview).

CAUSES

Major Untreatable Dementias

PRIMARY DEGENERATIVE DEMENTIA (DSM-III p 124, 290.xx)
(Alzheimer's and Pick's Diseases): Approx. 50% of all
dementias (5% of people over 65), but - usually a
diagnosis by exclusion. It is frequently over-
diagnosed. Usually begins insidiously in the 50's,
60's, or 70's and progresses relentlessly to death in
4-8 years. Ceaseless pacing and a shuffling gait are
common; social responses often remain intact until
very late. Look for cortical atrophy and enlarged
ventricles by CT scan. EEG is often normal for age
early on - a good screening test since it is often
abnormal with reversible causes of dementia (except
for general paresis and NPH). Histologically there
are senile placques, neurofibrillary tangles, and
neuronal granulovacuolar degeneration. Recent
evidence implicates primary degeneration of
cholinergic neurons of the basal forebrain,
particularly the nucleus basalis (Coyle et al, 1983).
There is an increased incidence in women (1.5:1),
first-degree relatives, and Down's syndrome.

Huntington's Chorea: Psychiatric symptoms, ranging from
neurotic to psychotic (including dementia), may
precede the chorea. Dementia always occurs
terminally. Autosomal dominant - so check family
history.

Parkinson's Disease: Depression and/or dementia in some
patients. L-Dopa relieves temporarily only.

Others: Progressive Supranuclear Palsy, spinocerebellar
degenerations, Parkinsonism-Dementia Complex of Guam,
SSPE, Creutzfeldt-Jakob Disease, herpes simplex
encephalitis, MS.

Treatable Forms of Dementia

MULTI-INFARCT DEMENTIA (DSM-III p 127, 290.4): 10% of
dementias. Differentiate from Primary Degenerative
Dementia by history of rapid onset and stepwise
deterioration in a patient in his 50's or early 60's
and by presence of focal neurological impairment.   EEG
may show focal abnormalities. Caused by multiple
thromboembolic episodes (numerous small cerebral
infarcts pathologically) in a patient with
atherosclerotic disease of the major vessels or
valvular disease of the heart. Hypertension is

usually present. Pseudobulbar phenomena are common:
emotional lability, dysarthria, dysphagia.
Controlling BP may help.

Normal Pressure Hydrocephalus (NPH): A "classic triad" of
gait ataxia, incontinence, and progressive dementia –
either idiopathic or following cerebral trauma,
hemorrhage, or infection. There is normal CSF
pressure but dilated ventricles by CT scan and pneumo-
encephalography. Confirm with isotope cisternography.
Treat with a lumboperitoneal or ventriculoatrial shunt –
55% show improvement.

DEMENTIA ASSOCIATED WITH ALCOHOLISM (DSM-III p 137, 291.2):
A diagnosis by exclusion – following many years of
heavy drinking. May be partly reversible with good
nutrition and abstinence.

Drug Intoxication: Common, particularly in the elderly
(too many meds, misunderstood instructions, etc).
Watch for major and minor tranquilizers, analgesics
(particularly phenacetin), digoxin, primidone,
diphenylhydantoin, methyldopa, and bromides.
Reevaluate and stop, if possible.

Brain Tumors: Primarily metastatic tumors (from lung and
breast) and meningiomas. Focal signs are usually
present except in frontal lobe. Get CSF pressure and
protein, EEG, and CT scan. EEG may be localizing.

Brain Trauma: Dementia is rare except for subdural
hematoma in the elderly – dementia, headache, and
drowsiness developing over weeks or months with or
without a history of trauma. Don't do LP. Get CT
scan, then arteriography (diagnostic). May be
reversible.

Infection: Any significant infection (eg, pneumonia, UTI)
can produce delirium and worsen a dementia in the
elderly. Dementia can be caused by brain abscess, CNS
syphilis (general paresis – serologic tests of blood
and CSF usually positive), and tuberculous and crypto-
coccal meningitis.

Metabolic Disorders: Most common are thyroid disorders –
hypothyroidism (dementia even with near normal hormone
levels; may be reversible; look for diffuse slowing on
EEG) and also hyperthyroidism ("apathetic thyrotoxicosis" – particularly in elderly). Electrolyte
imbalances are also common causes in the elderly – eg,
hypo- and hypernatremia and hypercalcemia. Suspect

Wilson's Disease if there are signs of liver failure, tremor, rigidity, and convulsions in a person under 40. Also consider Cushing's syndrome, hypoglycemia, and hyper- and hypoparathyroidism.

Disorders of heart, lung, liver, kidney: Particularly CHF, arrhythmias, SBE, chronic hypoxia and hypercapnia (eg, emphysema), hepatic encephalopathy, uremia, dialysis dementia.

Other: Malnutrition (particularly Vitamin B12 and folate deficiencies - check for pernicious anemia and combined system disease), toxins (eg, lead, mercury, nitrobenzenes, organophosphates), remote effects of carcinoma, SLE, epilepsy.

DIFFERENTIAL DIAGNOSIS

Normal aging may mimic mild dementia, particularly if the patient is stressed by environmental changes, social isolation, fatigue, or visual and hearing disorders (sensory deprivation). Many elderly will develop mild anxiety, depressive, or hypochondriacal disorders which mimic dementia but, with persistent questioning and encouragement, normal memory, orientation, etc. can be seen. Intellectual deterioration with schizophrenia is differentiated from dementia by a history of psychosis and social withdrawal and by the presence of a characteristic thought disorder. An amytal interview may help distinguish dementia from catatonic schizophrenia. In delirium there is an altered and fluctuating level of consciousness. Delirium and dementia frequently coexist but the delirium must clear before the diagnosis of dementia can be made.

A Major Depression is the most common cause of pseudodementia. Unlike the demented patient, these patients have a rapid, recent onset (family can usually date it), complain of a severe memory loss, which is usually mild when tested, have marked affective changes, emphasize their inabilities and failings, and frequently answer simple questions with "I don't know" (the demented patient usually attempts an answer). A temporary clearing during an amytal interview and the lack of a deteriorating course helps identify these patients. Consider a DST and CT scan (Grunhaus et al, 1983). They usually improve with antidepressants or ECT.

Don't mistake an aphasia due to a focal lesion for a dementia (although perhaps 10% of severely demented patients have a related aphasia).

TREATMENT

Supportive Treatment:

- Provide good physical care - eg, good nutrition, eye glasses, hearing aids, protection (eg, stairs, stoves, medication), etc.
- Keep in familiar settings, if possible. Surround with familiar objects; keep old friends engaged. Encourage the family's participation and understanding (Mace and Rabins, 1981).
- Keep the patient involved - through personal contact, frequent orientation (remind him of the day, of the time). Discuss the news with him. Use calendars, radio, TV. Structure daily activities - make them predictable.
- Help maintain patient's self-esteem. Treat like an adult. Plan towards his strengths. Be accepting, tolerant.
- Avoid dark, isolated settings; avoid overstimulation.

Symptomatic Treatment:

Psychiatric conditions require small doses of appropriate medication.

- Acute anxiety, restlessness, aggression: eg, haloperidol 0.5 mg PO TID; thioridazine, 25 mg PO TID-QID.
- Nonpsychotic anxiety: eg, diazepam 2 mg PO BID-TID; oxazepam 10 mg PO BID-TID.
- Depression: begin slowly and work up to - eg, imipramine 75-150 mg PO daily.
- Insomnia: for short periods only; use flurazepam 15 mg PO HS, or chlorpromazine 25-50 mg PO HS.

Specific Treatment:

- Identify and correct any treatable condition.
- No specific drug treatment for dementia has been found to be consistently useful although many are being investigated - eg, cerebral vasodilators, anti-coagulants, cerebral metabolic stimulants, stimulants, hyperbaric oxygen. Increasing central cholinergic activity may relieve some symptoms in a few patients with Primary Degenerative Dementia temporarily. Acetylcholine precursors (choline, 4 oz/day; lecithin 100 g/day - a large dose) may improve memory moderately in a few people, while acetylcholinesterase inhibitors (eg, physostigmine) show promise (Davis and Mohs, 1982).

REFERENCES

1. Coyle JT, Price DL, DeLong MR: Alzheimer's disease: a disorder of cortical cholinergic innervation. Science 219:1184, 1983.
2. Cummings JL, Benson DF: Dementia: A Clinical Approach. London, Butterworths, 1983.
3. Cummings JL, Benson DF, LoVerme S: Reversible dementia. JAMA 243:2434, 1980.
4. Davis KL, Mohs RC: Enhancement of memory processes in Alzheimer's disease with multiple-dose intravenous physostigmine. Am J Psychiat 139:1421, 1982.
5. Folstein MF, Folstein SE, McHugh PR: "Mini-mental state": a practical method for grading the mental state of patients for the clinician. J Psychiatr Res 12:189, 1975.
6. Grunhaus L, Dilsaver S, Grader JF, Carroll BJ: Depressive pseudodementia: a suggested diagnostic profile. Biolog Psychiat 18:215, 1983.
7. Heston LL, Mastri AR, Anderson E, White J: Dementia of the Alzheimer type. Arch Gen Psychiat 38:1085, 1981.
8. Mace NL, Rabins PV: The 36-Hour Day. Baltimore, Johns Hopkins Univ Pr, 1981.
9. Mayeux R, Rosen WG: The Dementias. New York, Raven Pr, 1983.
10. McAllister T: Overview: pseudodementia. Am J Psychiat 140:528, 1983.
11. McL. Black P: Normal-pressure hydrocephalus. Postgraduate Med 71, No 2: 57, 1982.
12. Naguib M, Levy R: Prediction of outcome in senile dementia - a computed tomography study. Brit J Psychiat 140:263, 1982.
13. Reifler BV, Larson E, Hanley R: Coexistence of cognitive impairment and depression in geriatric outpatients. Am J Psychiat 139:623, 1982.
14. Ron MA, Toone BK, Garralda ME, Lishman WA: Diagnostic accuracy in presenile dementia. Br J Psychiat 134:161, 1979.
15. Schneck MK, Reisberg B, Ferris SH: An overview of current concepts of Alzheimer's disease. Am J Psychiat 139:165, 1982.
16. Wells CE: Dementia, 2nd Ed. Philadelphia, F.A. Davis Co, 1977.
17. Wells CE: Pseudodementia. Am J Psychiatry 136:895, 1979.

Chapter 7

Suicidal and Assaultive Behaviors

THE SUICIDAL PATIENT

EPIDEMIOLOGY:

- Reported suicides in the USA - 28,000/yr (12/100,000).
- Suicide is under-reported - often listed as accidental.
- Attempted suicide:successful suicide ratio is 20:1.
- Suicide increases with age to peak at 60 years; 2nd leading cause of death among adolescents and college students.
- Completers 3:1 (male:female); attempters 3:1 (F:M).
- Most common attempt is by drug ingestion; most likely to be fatal is by shooting.

All clinicians will encounter suicidal patients. Many will not recognize them. Some of those patients will kill themselves.

IDENTIFYING THE POTENTIALLY SUICIDAL PATIENT

One fifth of suicides are unsuspected. Accurate prediction may be impossible (Pokorny, 1983). We must entertain the possibility when:

1. Suicide attempt: Patient seen in the ER, the medical ward, etc.
2. Overt or indirect suicide talk or threats: "You won't be bothered by me much longer."
3. Depressed or anxious mood due to a depression.
4. Significant recent loss: eg, spouse, job, self-esteem.
5. Unexpected change in behavior: making a will, buying a gun, giving away possessions, intense talks with friends.
6. Unexpected change in attitude: Suddenly cheerful, angry, or withdrawn.

ASSESSING SUICIDAL RISK

<u>Population Risk Factors</u>: Males, elderly, the socially
        isolated, whites, American Indians, policemen,
        psychiatrists.

Individual Risk Factors:
- Sense of <u>hopelessness</u>, helplessness, loneliness,
    exhaustion.
- <u>Past history of suicide attempts</u>, particularly serious
    attempts.
- Nature of past or present suicide attempts: eg, shooting
    or jumping more lethal than most ingestions or wrist
    cutting. Warning given? Help available at the time?
- Family history of suicide (Roy, 1983).
- Active use (abuse) of <u>alcohol</u> and drugs.
- Psychiatric illness, particularly:
    Major affective disorder - particularly with
        vegetative signs.
    Schizophrenia, particularly chronic, or with
        persecutory delusions or self-destructive command
        hallucinations.
    Psychoses due to organic brain syndromes.
    Alcoholism (suicide rate 50X norm - 25% of <u>all</u>
        suicides).
    Drug addiction (10% die by suicide).
    Personality disorders - particularly compulsive and
        borderline types.
- Widowed, divorced, separated, <u>single</u>, retired,
    <u>unemployed</u>.
- Impaired impulse control for any reason.
- Medical patients on renal dialysis.
- Failing health, particularly if previously independent.
- Family stresses or instability.
- A change in status - up or down.
- Recently experienced loss or rejection.
- Parental loss during childhood.
- Limited external support systems.

Other Risk Factors:
- Holidays, spring, anniversaries.
- Possible biochemical measures of suicide potential:
    decreased CSF 5-HIAA and increased MHPG (Brown et at,
    1982); positive DST (Targum et al, 1983).

ASSESSMENT PROCEDURE:

    <u>First</u>, build rapport during a supportive, non-
judgemental interview. If not volunteered, investigate
suicidal thoughts by asking questions of increasing
specificity: eg, "Have you been feeling sad?"; "Have you
thought of doing away with yourself?"; "How?"; etc. Asking

about suicide does not precipitate it. After a serious
attempt, wait until the patient is alert enough to
cooperate.

The following must be learned about all suicidal
patients:

1. The patient's intention - why does he want to die?
2. Is a suicide plan made? - the more specific the plan,
   the more likely the act.
3. Method - the more lethal the technique, the more serious
   the plan.
4. Presence of psychiatric or organic factors - eg,
   psychotic depression, thought disorder, sedative self-
   medication, organicity.
5. Determine the role of impulsivity vs premeditation.
6. Is the precipitating crisis resolving?
7. Take an "inventory of loss."
8. Does the patient have plans for the future?
9. Does the patient have caring family or other supports?

INITIATING APPROPRIATE TREATMENT

If the patient has pressing suicidal thoughts and/or
decreased impulse control coupled with several risk
factors, hospitalize, if only overnight. Be conservative.
Don't write patients off as "just manipulative" - all
statements of suicidal intent initially should be taken
seriously. A few manipulative suicide patients have
"accidentally" killed themselves after being denied
admission - 60% of successful suicides have had previous
suicide attempts. The most emotionally upset patient is
not necessarily the most suicidal. The suicidal state is
episodic, occasionally allowing a patient to be considerably less dangerous just hours after a serious suicide
attempt. Be very cautious of the patient who has trouble
considering any alternative to suicide.

A fundamental issue is whether or not to hospitalize.
A patient of lesser risk may be followed as an outpatient
if there is a reliable family to help monitor the patient -
assess that support. If the patient is not to be
hospitalized, definite and specific plans for follow-up
must be made with the patient and these must be clearly
understood by him. The decision to hospitalize should be
decisively but optimistically communicated to the patient.
Hospitalization should be involuntary if necessary. Assure
the patient's physical safety in the hospital through
appropriate "suicide precautions," eg, close supervision,
no isolation, no dangerous objects.

TREATMENT PRINCIPLES:

1. Identify psychiatric or medical conditions requiring definitive treatment.
   a. Treat psychotic depressions with tricyclics and an antipsychotic. If the patient is determinedly suicidal, use ECT rather than wait for a medication response.
   b. Use antipsychotics with schizophrenic patients.
   c. Phenothiazines and benzodiazepines may be briefly useful with the agitated patient.
2. Develop a therapeutic alliance with the patient. Be concerned and accepting. Attempt to understand why the patient wants to die. Allow him to express anger, "unacceptable" thoughts, and feelings of rejection and hopelessness. These patients often feel misunderstood and trapped but unable to ask for help.
3. Suicidal patients are usually ambivalent about death and often don't know why they are trying to kill themselves. Point out that ambivalence to them - show them evidence of their desire to live. Be hopeful. Be definite. Make specific plans with and for the patient. Appeal to his mature rather than his regressive side.
4. The patients are often bewildered and have a narrowed focus of thought - deal with reality issues.
5. Don't minimize the seriousness of a suicide attempt to the patient.
6. Never agree to hold a suicide plan in confidence.
7. Help the patient to grieve over losses.
8. Do not explain away the patient's symptoms - eg, "I'd feel the same way."
9. Use community resources. Involve the family and significant others actively in treatment. Use family therapy when appropriate. Actively try to reduce social isolation and withdrawal. Help make changes in the patient's environment where it is pathological.
10. Many suicides occur during periods of improvement from depression - eg, the first 3-6 months after hospital discharge. Monitor closely during holidays.
11. Be active but insist that the patient ultimately take responsibility for his own life.
12. Tricyclics, MAO inhibitors, and many sedative-hypnotics have serious overdose potential. Some depressed outpatients store medication so keep careful track of medication prescribed.

Theoretical explanations of suicide include the loss of a sense of identity with the social group (Durkheim), hostility turned against the self (Freud), a "cry for

help," and a reflection of biologic, psychiatric
conditions.

THE VIOLENT PATIENT

Human aggression has complex and uncertain biological
(androgens and the limbic system), psychosocial, and
cultural roots.   Prediction of violence is difficult.
Anyone can become violent yet some groups are at risk:
young males 15-25, urban, black, violent cultural sub-
groups, alcoholics. The best individual predictors of
violent behavior are:

1. A past history of violence
2. Active use of alcohol
3. Neglect and physical abuse as a child

The "classic triad" of enuresis, firesetting, and cruelty
to animals as a child is perhaps less predictive of adult
violence than childhood fighting, temper tantrums, truancy,
and interpersonal difficulties (Justice et al, 1974).

MENTAL DISORDERS WITH ASSOCIATED VIOLENT BEHAVIOR:

Although most mentally ill are not dangerous, some
patients present an increased risk.

1. Schizophrenia, paranoid and catatonic types - particularly with command hallucinations or in patients who
   drink.
2. Alcohol and drug abuse - particularly PCP and amphetamines (either when "high" or during paranoid
   withdrawal states); also LSD, "downers," cocaine.
3. Organic brain syndromes - particularly with confusion or
   decreased impulse control; eg, drugs in the elderly,
   hypoglycemia, CNS infections, anoxia, metabolic
   acidosis.
4. Acute psychotic states of any origin.
5. The mentally retarded; XYY karyotype - possibly.
6. Attention deficit disorder with hyperactivity, in adults.

But, most violence is not related to mental illness.

SEVERAL RECOGNIZABLE PATTERNS OF VIOLENCE

1. Chronic, aggressive, self-aggrandizing life style - seen
   with antisocial personality disorder and thus
   associated with drug and alcohol abuse, onset in
   youth, delinquency and adult crime, truancy and school
   failure. Patients fight frequently and are
   "constantly in trouble."

2. Episodic violence - explosive rages with little provo-
   cation, daily to several times/yr, brief, occasional
   amnesia for event and remorse about it. A confusing
   group of clinical presentations that may overlap or be
   synonymous (see Leicester, 1982).
       If violence is directed: consider (1)
   INTERMITTENT EXPLOSIVE DISORDER (DSM-III p 295,
   312.34) - usually males with history of violent
   outbursts, family history of violence, neurological
   soft signs, abnormal EEGs, normal between episodes;
   (2) Episodic Dyscontrol Syndrome (Mark et al, 1970) -
   history of violence, pathological intoxication,
   impulsive sexual behavior, and frequent traffic
   violations; or (3) rages in borderline or histrionic
   personality disorders.
       If violence poorly directed: consider temporal
   lobe epilepsy (get NP leads; see Pincus, 1981),
   pathological intoxication.
3. Single extremely violent outburst in normally compliant
   person - ISOLATED EXPLOSIVE DISORDER (DSM-III p 297,
   312.35). Often in an overcontrolled, inadequate,
   introverted personality under stress. Usually a
   surprise.

EVALUATING THREATS OF VIOLENCE

    Take all thoughts or threats of violence seriously.
Assess risk factors.
    What is the patient's current mental state - can he
control his impulses and rage? Does he feel under great
tension and fear losing control? Is there an intended
victim? Is the victim covertly provoking the attack?
Specific plans made? Sadistic fantasies present? Weapons
available? Patient armed (always check)? Family support
system present?

MANAGEMENT OF THE VIOLENT PATIENT

1. First decide if patient is acutely out of control. If
   so, treat immediately with restraint and medication,
   not talk.
2. Approach an unfamiliar patient cautiously and from a
   position of strength (help available, open door). If
   talking appears useful, try, but set clear limits
   during interview. Establish physical controls if
   patient can't maintain but emphasize their temporary,
   helping nature. If patient arrives in restraints,
   don't remove until rapport established and some
   evaluation done - however, many patients do better
   without restraints. Restraints may increase agitation
   and cause hyperthermia. If force is needed to subdue,

3. Medication:
   use overwhelming force - one person to each limb.
   Don't take chances.

3. Medication:
   For the majority of acutely agitated patients:
      haloperidol 5-10 mg IM every 45 minutes until calm
      (maximum 40 mg/24 hr - occasionally more).
   For immediate control (watch for respiratory
      depression): diazepam 5-10 mg IV given over 2
      minutes.
   Has patient taken CNS depressants or is a primary
      medical condition responsible for behavior? - If so,
      hold meds and observe. ECT can control psychotic
      violence.
4. If patient is threatening and agitated but not wild,
   treat with respect - be civil, direct, confident,
   reassuring. Don't challenge or provoke the patient.
   Eliminate red tape. Violent patients are often
   frightened - find out why and of what.
5. Determine etiology of violence. Is a mental illness
   present? Drugs involved (get urine screen)? Are
   there identifiable environmental precipitants? Expect
   to treat the psychotic patient with more direct
   intervention. If additional information is needed,
   consider an interview with family members present.
6. Most patients can be "talked down" with support, understanding (and medication) - however, hospitalize
   involuntarily if necessary. Is this really a criminal
   matter and should the police be involved instead?

ONGOING CARE

1. Teach patient to recognize early signs of increasing
   anger and to develop ways to discharge tension.
2. Help patient to develop a support system and to learn to
   control environmental stresses. Maintain a channel of
   communication with the potentially violent patient -
   be available by phone.
3. Treat psychosis and seizures with appropriate medication. Carbamazepine (Tegretol) may be particularly
   useful for seizure-like outbursts. Benzodiazepines
   can be useful during times of stress but paradoxical
   rages may occur in some patients. Some explosive,
   aggressive patients respond to lithium, some hyperactive adults may benefit from stimulants, and brain-
   damaged or mentally retarded patients may improve with
   propranolol (Ratey et al, 1983).
4. Psychosurgery may be useful in extreme cases.

REFERENCES

1. Brown GL, Ebert MH, Goyer PF, Jimerson DC, Klein WJ, Bunney WE, Goodwin FK: Aggression, suicide, and serotonin: relationships to CSF amine metabolites. Am J Psychiat 139:741, 1982.
2. Jacobs D: Evaluation and management of the violent patient in emergency settings. Psychiat Clin N Am 6:259, June 1983.
3. Jacobs D: Evaluation and care of suicidal behavior in emergency settings. Int'l J Psychiat in Med 12:295, 1982-83.
4. Justice B, Justice R, Kraft I: Early-warning signs of violence. Am J Psychiat 131:457, 1974.
5. Kovacs M, Beck AT, Weissman A: The communication of suicidal intent: a reexamination. Arch Gen Psychiat 33:198, 1976.
6. Leicester J: Temper tantrums, epilepsy, and episodic dyscontrol. Brit J Psychiat 141:262, 1982.
7. Mark VH, Ervin FR: Violence and the Brain. New York, Harper & Row, 1970.
8. Monahan J: The prediction of violent behavior: towards a second generation of theory and policy. Am J Psychiat 141:10, 1984.
9. Pincus JH: Violence and epilepsy (editorial). NEJM 305:696, 1981.
10. Pokorny AD: Prediction of suicide in psychiatric patients. Arch Gen Psychiat 40:249, 1983.
11. Ratey JJ, Morrill R, Oxenkrug G: Use of propranolol for provoked and unprovoked episodes of rage. Am J Psychiat 140:1356, 1983.
12. Roy A: Family history of suicide. Arch Gen Psychiat 40:971, 1983.
13. Targum SD, Rosen L, Capodanno AE: The dexamethasone suppression test in suicidal patients with unipolar depression. Am J Psychiat 140:877, 1983.

Chapter 8

Anxiety Disorders

Anxiety is ubiquitous; anxiety disorders are not. Anxiety is an unpleasant and unjustified sense of apprehension often accompanied by physiological symptoms, while anxiety disorder connotes significant distress and dysfunction due to the anxiety. An anxiety disorder may be characterized by only anxiety, or it may display another symptom such as a phobia or an obsession and present anxiety when the primary symptom is resisted. Fear is also universal and can produce the symptom picture of acute anxiety states yet, in contrast to anxiety, the cause is obvious and understandable. A feature common to all of the anxiety disorders is the unpleasant and unnatural quality of the symptoms (anxiety, phobia, obsession) - they are ego-alien or ego-dystonic.

CHRONIC, MILD ANXIETY

Tension, irritability, apprehension, and mild distractibility are common (particularly in medical and psychiatric patients), often related to environmental factors, and treated with supportive and reality-oriented therapy. Medications are of little value chronically while iatrogenic addiction is a serious problem. Environmentally induced, short-lived, mild anxiety (ADJUSTMENT DISORDER WITH ANXIOUS MOOD, DSM-III p 301, 309.24) usually resolves with the disappearance of the stress.

CHRONIC, MODERATELY SEVERE ANXIETY

A diagnosis of GENERALIZED ANXIETY DISORDER (Anxiety Neurosis) (DSM-III p 232, 300.02) is made with more severe, chronic symptoms (longer than 6 months) including autonomic responses (palpitations, diarrhea, cold clammy extremities, sweating, urinary frequency), insomnia, fatigue, sighing, trembling, and/or marked apprehension. Secondary depression is common. Usually no obvious etiologic stress is found, but look anyway. Psychotherapy helps (40% of patients). Encourage self-reliance and maintenance of productive activity. Train the patient in relaxation techniques; eg, biofeedback, meditation, self-hypnosis. Use benzodiazepines sparingly (diazepam, 5 mg, PO, TID-QID, or 10 mg HS) and for short periods only (weeks) - patients are at risk for addiction. Over 50% of patients become asymptomatic with time (months, years) but the rest retain a significant degree of impairment (Noyes et al, 1980). Help the patient understand the chronic nature of the illness and the likelihood of having to live with some symptoms.

ACUTE ANXIETY — PANIC ATTACKS

A PANIC DISORDER (DSM-III p 230, 300.01) has dramatic, acute symptoms lasting minutes to hours, is self-limited, and occurs in patients with or without chronic anxiety. Symptoms are perceived by the patient as medical and are characteristic of strong autonomic discharge - heart pounding, chest pains, trembling, choking, abdominal pain, sweating, dizziness - as well as disorganization, confusion, dread, and often a sense of impending doom or terror. Attacks often are initiated by crowds or stressful locations, may be repeated several times daily, weekly, or monthly, and often disappear for months at a time (but may become chronic). A typical panic attack can be produced by the intravenous infusion of sodium lactate in patients with panic disorder, but not in normals.

Like other anxiety conditions, it runs in families. It often is associated with major depression and/or alcoholism and it occurs more frequently in women (2:1), particularly those who have had a disturbed childhood and early difficulty separating from their parents (separation anxiety disorder). In its milder forms, panic disorder tends to grade into the Generalized Anxiety Disorder clinically (although it appears to be a distinct disorder). Patients often receive the "million dollar workup" for angina, thyrotoxicosis, or abdominal complaints. Effective treatment exists.

1. Supportive psychotherapy is of use acutely but does not correct the condition or prevent relapses.
2. Tricyclic antidepressants (imipramine) or MAOIs (phenelzine) are specific treatments which usually are effective more quickly and at lower doses (eg, imipramine 75-100 mg/day) than those needed for the antidepressant effect - not yet approved by the FDA.
3. Benzodiazepines are of moderate use acutely (chlordia-zepoxide 10-25 mg, PO, TID-QID; diazepam 5-10 mg, PO, TID-QID).

4. Beta-adrenergic blockers (propranolol) may be of value
   in controlling symptoms (particularly in patients with
   associated MVPS) but are not standard treatment.
   Clonidine (an antihypertensive drug) may effectively
   control panic attacks in some people (Ko et al, 1983).

ANXIETY WITH SPECIFIC FEARS — PHOBIC DISORDERS

Phobias are fears which are persistent and intense,
are out of proportion to the stimulus, make little sense
even to the sufferer, lead to avoidance of the feared
object or situation, and when sufficiently distressful or
disabling, are termed a PHOBIC DISORDER. Common, mild,
irrational fears (of the dark, heights, snakes) receive no
diagnosis. Phobias may wax and wane over months or years,
continue for decades, and may gradually resemble a
depressive disorder. They tend to generalize during their
developing stages - eg, fear of a store generalizes to the
street in front of the store and then to the entire
shopping area.

Up to 7% of the population may have a phobic disorder
in some circumstances yet in less than 1% is it significantly disabling. The majority begin suddenly in women
from stable families and of ages 15-30. Anxiety with
ruminations may dominate the day to day picture or anxiety
may occur only when the phobic object is encountered
directly. Relief occurs with escape, thus reinforcing the
avoidance pattern - a vicious circle. Phobics are at risk
to abuse alcohol and drugs as self-medication. Three
subtypes have been identified (although perhaps the more
important distinction is whether or not the phobia is
accompanied by a panic disorder):

AGORAPHOBIA (DSM-III p 226, 300.21 and .22):

Multiple phobias with chronic anxiety and occasionally
panic attacks. Specifically fears of open and/or closed
spaces, crowded places, unfamiliar places, and being
alone. Many other fears and hypochondriacal concerns
may be present, as well as multiple other symptoms
including fainting, obsessional thoughts, depersonalization (feel unreal, detached), and derealization (feel
surroundings are unreal). Patients with significant
panic attacks may have developed their agoraphobia as an
extension of a panic disorder - ie, unpredictable panic
attacks cause them to avoid public places for fear of
having an attack (anticipatory anxiety). Constitutes
approximately 50% of the phobic patients - the most
disabling type. Women:men = 2:1. 20% of agoraphobics
have a similarly affected relative.

SOCIAL PHOBIA (DSM-III p 227, 300.23):

Fear of public speaking, using public lavatories,
blushing, eating in public. Some patients exhibit
marked general anxiety, others very little. Patient
controls by avoidance - can be socially crippling.
Don't mistake for the social withdrawal of some
personality disorders, depressions, schizophrenia, or
paranoid states.

SIMPLE PHOBIAS (DSM-III p 228, 300.29):

Monophobias - of animals, thunderstorms, needles, etc.
Usually begin in childhood, are more frequent among
women, and have few associated symptoms or syndromes.

TREATMENT: Twofold.

1. Behavior therapy - primarily with simple phobias and
perhaps social phobias, but also agoraphobia without
panic attacks. Key to treatment is exposure to the
feared object. Systematic desensitization (by
reciprocal inhibition) utilizes a graded hierarchy of
frightening stimuli allowing the patient to "work up" to
facing the phobic object. In flooding the patient faces
the feared object or situation directly while with
implosion the exposure is to the idea of the object or a
vivid account of the "terrible" consequences produced by
the object. Both exposures usually require and are
enhanced by support and/or antianxiety medication.

2. Medication. Minor tranquilizers are used temporarily to
help the patient confront the phobia. Beta blockers
(eg, propranolol) can be used occasionally to help
control incapacitating autonomic symptoms (eg, before a
speech). If the course is complicated by panic attacks,
consider tricyclic antidepressants (imipramine 25-50 mg,
PO, HS-TID) or MAO inhibitors (phenelzine 15 mg, PO,
TID). Once the panic attacks are controlled with
medication, an agoraphobic often needs supportive
exposure to the feared situations (without experiencing
panic) before the phobia is resolved.

DIFFERENTIAL DIAGNOSIS OF ANXIETY STATES

The various anxiety disorders are mimicked by other
psychiatric conditions as well as by a number of medical
illnesses. Always rule out an anxious depression
(depressive symptoms appear first and usually predominate -
be suspicious of anxiety that first appears after age 30).

Alcohol and drug abuse (chronic hypnotic-sedative withdrawal, amphetamine use, caffeinism) are very common primary problems in patients presenting with uncomplicated anxiety. Numerous unexplained physical complaints, with or without frequent operations, suggest Somatization Disorder. Anxiety is often prominent in schizophrenia and in borderline and histrionic personality disorders, while an acute schizophrenic episode may present as a panic attack (with disordered thinking). Hyperventilation Syndrome (HVS) may be a separate syndrome - a vicious cycle developed in susceptible persons: anxiety causes hyperventilation causes respiratory alkalosis causes vasoconstriction causes symptoms (light-headedness, paresthesias, carpopedal spasms) causes anxiety - treat with rebreathing, education.

Medical conditions (most commonly cardiac disorders) may also mimic anxiety states, although often they produce no sense of apprehension or foreboding. If suggestive physical symptoms accompany anxiety, remember:

1. Abnormal EKG's and heart sounds help identify cardiac symptoms (chest pain, palpitations) due to angina pectoris, prolapse of the mitral valve (mid- or late systolic click), and cardiac arrhythmias (eg, PAT). Mitral valve prolapse syndrome (MVPS) accompanies 20-30% of patients with agoraphobia - the anxiety surrounding the sudden heart symptoms may lead to agoraphobia in susceptible persons.
2. The apprehension and dyspnea associated with bronchial asthma or COLD ("pink puffers") usually has accompanying wheezing or characteristic spirometric and radiographic features.
3. Acute Intermittent Porphyria - anxiety with abdominal focus; look for fever, leukocytosis, pain in extremities, prior drug exposure, elevated urine porphobilinogen; Watson-Schwartz Test is positive.
4. Characteristic findings usually occur with duodenal ulcer (bleeding, relief of pain with food, persistent crater by X-ray, suggestive gastric analysis) and ulcerative colitis (bloody diarrhea, fever, weight loss, sigmoidoscopic findings) but without them, differentiation is sometimes difficult. Internal hemorrhage may be accompanied by pain and restlessness - the picture develops quickly.
5. The vertiginous, anxious patient with Meniere's Disease also has deafness, tinnitus, and nystagmus during the attack.

If there are no localizing features to the acute attack or if the anxiety is chronic, consider:

6. Hypoglycemia - at times indistinguishable from chronic or acute anxiety; obtain blood glucose at the time of the episode; 5 hr GTT.
7. Hyperthyroidism - anxiety symptoms occur with rapid onset type; skin warm and moist rather than cold and clammy; look for exophthalmos; get T3, T4; check for goiter; consider TRH stimulation test.
8. Pheochromocytoma - anxiety attacks with hypertension; visual blurring, headache, perspiration, palpitations; get 24 hr urinary VMA or free catecholamines.

Other medical conditions can mimic the anxiety syndromes: intracranial tumors, menstrual irregularities, hypothyroidism, hyper- and hypoparathyroidism, post-concussion syndrome, psychomotor epilepsy, Cushing's Disease. Appropriate tests help differentiate.

ANXIETY WITH OBSESSIONS AND COMPULSIONS

OBSESSIVE COMPULSIVE DISORDER (DSM-III p 234, 300.30)
(Obsessive Compulsive Neurosis)

Obsessions are repetitive ideas, images, and impulses which intrude upon a patient who feels powerless to stop them. They are usually unpleasant, always unwanted, and may be frightening or violent (eg, the impulse to leap before a car; the thought of a friend being harmed). The patient can ruminate endlessly ("Did I lock the door?") and may develop rituals or compulsions (counting, touching) to ward off unwanted happenings or to satisfy an obsession (eg, an obsession with dirt leading to handwashing rituals). Compulsions are thus obsessions made manifest and occur in 75% of obsessives. Their performance relieves the anxiety of the obsession temporarily. The thinking is often magical ("My son won't have an accident if I stamp each foot 30 times.") and the patient is generally aware of this.

The disorder is uncommon and chronic, with some spontaneous cures. There is increased concordance for obsessions in monozygotes and often a family history for obsessional disorder. First symptoms usually occur by the early 20's, may begin suddenly or slowly, and often have an episodic course. Often the clinical picture is dominated by the rituals, requiring them to be treated directly.

DIFFERENTIAL: Obsessive-compulsive problems are common in serious psychiatric illnesses. 20% of serious depressions have obsessive symptoms - major symptoms and family history help separate - treatment may be identical. Schizophrenics have bizarre obsessions and are usually comfortable with

them. Organic Mental Disorders may present early with
obsessions and compulsions.

TREATMENT:

    There are no certain cures. Behavior therapy
techniques appear the most useful: eg, interrupting the
performance of a compulsion (response prevention), shouting
to stop obsessional thoughts (thought stopping), or
application of aversive techniques. Rituals respond better
to treatment than obsessions, with the treatment of choice
being exposure to the dreaded situation while preventing
the performance of the ritual. If a ritual is coupled with
a depressed mood, exposure and antidepressants can be
markedly successful (Marks et al, 1980). Tricyclic antidepressants (clomipramine) also may be effective with some
obsessionals, even without prominent anxiety or depressive
symptoms. Psychosurgery helps the unusual, very chronic,
and very disabled patient.

REFERENCES

1. Amies PL, Gelder MG, Shaw PM: Social phobia: a
    comparative clinical study. Brit J Psychiat 142:174,
    1983.
2. Ananth J: Clomipramine in obsessive-compulsive
    disorder: a review. Psychosomatics 24:723, 1983.
3. Kantor JS, Zitrin CM, Zeldis SM: Mitral valve prolapse
    syndrome in agoraphobic patients. Am J Psychiat
    137:467, 1980.
4. Ko GN, Elsworth JD, Roth RH, Rifkin BG, Leigh H,
    Redmond E: Panic-induced elevation of plasma MHPG
    levels in phobic-anxious patients. Arch Gen Psychiat
    40:425, 1983.
5. Leckman JF, Weissman MM, Merikangas KR, Pauls DL,
    Prusoff BA: Panic disorder and major depression. Arch
    Gen Psychiat 40:1055, 1983.
6. Liebowitz MR, Klein DF: Differential diagnosis and
    treatment of panic attacks and phobic states. Ann Rev
    Med 32:583, 1981.
7. Mavissakalian M, Michelson L: Tricyclic antidepressants
    in obsessive-compulsive disorder. J Nerv Ment Dis
    171:301, 1983.
8. Mawson D, Marks IM, Ramm L: Clomipramine and exposure
    for chronic obsessive-compulsive rituals. Brit J
    Psychiat 140:11, 1982.
9. Noyes R, Clancy J, Hoenk PR, Slymen DJ: The prognosis
    of anxiety neurosis. Arch Gen Psychiat 37:173, 1980.

10. Sarwer-Foner GJ: Psychotherapeutic management of the severely anxious patient. Am J Psychotherapy 36:318, 1982.
11. Steketee G, Foa EB, Grayson JB: Recent advances in the behavioral treatment of obsessive-compulsives. Arch Gen Psychiat 39:1365, 1982.
12. Stern R, Cobb J: Phenomenology of obsessive-compulsive neurosis. Brit J Psychiat 132:233, 1978.
13. Tanna VT, Penningrowth RP, Woolson RF: Propranolol in anxiety neurosis. Compr Psychiat 18:319, 1977.
14. Tippin J, Henn FA: Modified leukotomy in the treatment of intractable obsessional neurosis. Am J Psychiat 139:1601, 1982.
15. Torgersen S: Genetic factors in anxiety disorders. Arch Gen Psychiat 40:1085, 1983.

Chapter 9

Dissociative Disorders

These are uncommon conditions, most of which had previously been classified as forms of hysterical neurosis, dissociative type.

AMNESIA

Organic processes (usually involving the temporal lobes) account for the majority of cases of significant memory loss in adults. These processes include intoxication or withdrawal from drugs or alcohol, various dementias, acute or chronic metabolic conditions (eg, hypoglycemia, hepatic encephalopathy), brain trauma (ie, postconcussive amnesia), brain tumors (particularly in the temporal lobes), cerebrovascular accidents, epilepsy (particularly temporal lobe epilepsy), and various degenerative or infectious CNS diseases. Transient Global Amensia (TGA) is a well-known, self-limited, massive loss of memory in middleaged or elderly patients due to a variety of organic causes. It always must be differentiated from psychological amnesia.

Loss of memory due primarily to psychological causes is PSYCHOGENIC AMNESIA (DSM-III p 253, 300.12). Although the amnesia may affect all memory, usually there is sudden anterograde loss for discrete categories of information following a severe physical or psychosocial stress. It occurs most frequently in women in their teens or 20's, or in men during the stress of war. The patient often appears confused and puzzled during the attack but recovery is usually rapid, spontaneous, and complete.

If the patient, in the context of a severe memory loss and usually following a major stress, leaves home and assumes a new identity, he has PSYCHOGENIC FUGUE (DSM-III p 255, 300.13). He is usually unaware of his previous (real) identity and appears to function relatively well in

his new role. The return of old memories and the old
identity is usually abrupt but may not occur for days,
weeks, or months (or longer).

The differential diagnosis of both conditions
includes:

1. Various organic conditions (see above).
2. Psychiatric conditions - Amnesia may often accompany
   severe depressive or anxiety states. Somnambulism may
   superficially resemble some fugues but has marked
   clouding of consciousness.
3. Malingering and secondary gain in patients with
   antisocial personality disorder.

Evaluate these patients with a careful history and
physical exam, liver enzymes, blood alcohol level and drug
screen, and skull X-ray. Further evaluation may include a
CAT scan and a sleep deprived EEG with NP leads. Are old
skills preserved during the attack (uncommon in organic
conditions)? Is there obvious secondary gain? Is there a
personal or family history for mental illness or epilepsy?
A diagnostic test in some cases is the amytal interview -
organic patients usually become more confused while
patients with psychological amnesia may have a return of
memory.

MULTIPLE PERSONALITY (DSM-III p 257, 300.14)

Patients with this dramatic disorder (eg, The Three
Faces of Eve) feel that they have at least two (and
sometimes many) complete personalities within themselves.
One of the personalities is usually dominant yet any one of
them may dominate from time to time. The patient's
behavior is consistent with whatever personality is in
"control" at that moment. Each different personality is
usually (but not always) aware of the presence of the
others.

This poorly understood psychiatric condition tends to
be chronic and may be a form of self-hypnosis. Some cases
have been felt to be hypnotic states inadvertently produced
by the treating physician. Considered rare, some experts
suggest that it may be more common, in disguised forms,
among patients with the more flamboyant personality
disorders, somatization disorder, and schizophrenia (Bliss,
1980 and 1983).

DEPERSONALIZATION DISORDER (DSM-III p 259, 300.60)

These patients experience periods during which they have a strong and unpleasant sense of their own unreality (depersonalization), often coupled with a sense that the environment is also unreal (derealization). The patient may feel mechanical and separated from his own thoughts, emotions, and self-identity. Although many people transiently experience this phenomenon in a mild form, the experience for those receiving a clinical diagnosis is much more intense. It occurs suddenly (often during relaxation following stress), usually in persons in their teens or 20's, may last for minutes, hours, or days, and then gradually disappears. It may return many times over the years.

Treatment has been of little value. Rule out the symptom of depersonalization that may accompany psychiatric disorders (eg, schizophrenia, depression, anxiety disorders, and histrionic personality disorder) and organic conditions (eg, OBS, temporal lobe epilepsy, drug and alcohol use, brain tumor).

REFERENCES

1. Akhtar S, Brenner I: Differential diagnosis of fugue-like states. J Clin Psychiat 40:381, September, 1979.
2. Bliss EL: Multiple personalities: a report of 14 cases with implications for schizophrenia and hysteria. Arch Gen Psychiat 37:1388, 1980.
3. Bliss EL, Larson EM, Nakashima SR: Auditory hallucinations and schizophrenia. J Nerv Ment Dis 171:30, 1983.
4. Confer WN, Ables BS: Multiple Personality: Etiology, Diagnosis and Treatment. New York, Human Sciences Pr., 1983.
5. Coryell W: Multiple personality and primary affective disorder. J Nerv Ment Dis 171:388,1983.
6. Kluft RP. An introduction to multiple personality disorder. Psychiat Annals 14:19, January, 1984.
7. Nausieda PA, Sherman IC: Long-term prognosis in transient global amnesia. JAMA 241:392, 1979.
8. Whitty CWM, Zangwill OL: Amnesia: Clinical, Psychological, and Medicolegal Aspects. London, Butterworths, 1977.

Chapter 10

Grief and the Dying Patient

Everyone endures personal losses. Everyone dies. Many people suffer chronic illnesses. Physicians often attend at all of these events and need to recognize normal and abnormal human responses to loss (grief reaction and unresolved grief), illness, and death.

GRIEF REACTION

NORMAL GRIEF:

Symptoms:

UNCOMPLICATED BEREAVEMENT (DSM-III p 333, V62.82) (grief, mourning) is a normal response to a significant loss (of spouse, parent, child - but also of health, limb, career, savings, status, etc). Expect to see it with major losses - be alert for future problems if the patient doesn't grieve (although 30% of widows mourn briefly and very little). If one is aware of an impending loss, often mourning begins long before the loss actually occurs (anticipatory grief). Symptoms associated with divorce may also be coded as MARITAL PROBLEM (DSM-III p 333, V61.10).

Recognize grief by restlessness, distractibility, disorganization, preoccupation, "numbness," feelings of sadness, apathy, crying, anxious pining, a need to talk about the dead, and intense mental pain during the days, weeks, and months after a loss. Somatic distress is common and includes generalized weakness, a tightness in the throat, choking, shortness of breath, palpitations, headaches, and GI complaints. Do not be surprised if the patient displays marked but short-lived irritability, hostility, or anger towards you, others, or the dead (you didn't "do enough"; they don't "care enough," he died, etc). This often alternates with listlessness, social withdrawal, depression, and feelings of guilt (about that

which was left undone or all that could have been done
differently). Typically, patients are preoccupied with
their loss. They think about the dead constantly,
continually review past experiences, visit the grave, and
may even briefly deny the death.

25-35% of patients have symptoms suggesting a major
depression: anorexia, insomnia, impaired memory, suicidal
thoughts, and hopelessness. 10% have delusional thoughts
and hallucinations. Be careful not to "over-read"
temporary bizarre behavior in the bereaved. Some patients
develop psychophysiologic disorders, hypochondriasis, major
anxiety symptoms, or phobias. A few begin to drink too
much, some deteriorate physically, and major psychiatric
illnesses (eg, acute schizophrenia) may be precipitated in
those predisposed (eg, positive family history).

Course:

All these symptoms are usually short-lived. Patients
suffering acute, unanticipated losses may have a brief
period of shock and disbelief but then they typically begin
to grieve, although occasionally mourning develops slowly
over days or weeks. Symptoms usually peak after 1-4 weeks
and then gradually disappear but brief relapses are
frequent as situations remind the patient of his loss.
Resolution occurs over 6-12 weeks but may require as much
as 1-2 years. Transient symptoms may reappear at special
times (eg, anniversaries, holidays).

UNRESOLVED GRIEF:

Loss not dealt with through a normal mourning process
may produce chronic symptoms.

- Prolonged Grief: Grief develops into a chronic, low
    level depression in some. Lowered self-esteem and
    guilt tend to be prominent.
- Delayed Grief: The patient who doesn't grieve at the
    time of a loss is at risk for later depression, social
    withdrawal, anxiety disorders, panic attacks, overt or
    covert self-destructive behavior, alcoholism, and
    psychophysiologic syndromes. Chronic anger and
    hostility, marked emotional inhibition, or distorted
    interpersonal relationships also may be displayed.
    Unresolved grief may be an unsuspected cause of
    psychiatric disability in many people - always inquire
    about a past history of significant losses.
- Distorted Grief: Exaggerated (bizarre, hysterical,
    euphoric or psychotic-like) reactions occur in a few
    patients which have the effect of postponing the

normal grieving process. Alternately, the patient may present with physical complaints (eg, pain or "chronic illness behavior") and be mistaken for having a primary medical problem.

Persons at risk for developing an abnormal grief reaction include those who:

1. Received little support or understanding from others following their loss (eg, abortion, suicide, death of an illicit lover).
2. Are social isolates - either "psychological loners" or those without family or friends nearby. The presence of multiple strong supports help truncate the mourning process.
3. Are inhibited, compulsive, or uncomfortable with any form of emotion.
4. Have experienced multiple recent losses or a sudden, severe, unexpected loss.
5. Have unresolved past losses.
6. Had ambivalent feelings about the deceased and have reacted to the death with guilt.

TREATMENT:

Encouraging satisfactory mourning is an important activity for the physician.

- Encourage mourning. Say it is OK. Say it is important and necessary. Explain that the anguish he undoubtedly will experience during this process is essential and curative. However, do not force the patient - let him set the pace.
- Help the patient identify and experience his emotions - sadness, hopelessness, despair, anxiety, fear, anger. Assure him that these are normal, expected, and understandable. Do not be embarrassed by these emotions yourself.
- Help the patient review his loss. Be an active listener. Ask for a description of the deceased - ask for particulars, details, shared intimacies, etc. Develop a supportive relationship with the patient during this process.
- See the patient frequently. Be interested. Be available, particularly over time. Recognize and tolerate relapses. Be alert to the presence of anniversaries.
- Do not use medication to attenuate normal grief - help the patient work through the grief instead. Sleeping medication may be useful. If anxiety or restlessness is excessive, consider a temporary use of minor tranquilizers (eg, diazepam 5 mg PO TID) as therapy is

begun. Treat a major depression or psychosis.
- Work with the family. Help develop a sympathetic support
  system. Mourners are social outcasts - help decrease
  the "social isolation of the bereaved." Self-help
  groups can be very valuable (eg, groups of parents who
  have lost a child, etc).
- Keep the mourner "involved in life" - slowly at first,
  but insist on increasing independence.

POST-TRAUMATIC STRESS DISORDER

If a patient suffers an exceptionally severe and
unusual loss or stress (eg, rape, car accident, fire,
natural disaster, prison camp, etc), he may develop a
recognizable clinical syndrome which includes intrusive
ideas of the event, a reliving of the feelings experienced
at the time, an emotional blunting which can impair
interpersonal relationships and day to day functioning, and
acute episodes of anxiety and depression. This pattern has
much in common with normal and unresolved grief. If the
reaction lasts less than 6 months it is considered POST-
TRAUMATIC STRESS DISORDER, ACUTE (DSM-III p 236, 308.30)
and, if it lasts longer than 6 months or doesn't begin
until at least 6 months after the event, it becomes
CHRONIC or DELAYED (DSM-III p 236, 309.81).

Treat as you would a more typical grief reaction. The
rape victim needs special and sensitive care (often in the
ER) after the assault, for psychiatric as well as legal
reasons (Falk, 1977). Many of her other interpersonal
relationships may have been altered by that episode. Work
with the family - often the married victim needs to
establish a new equilibrium with her husband.

THE DYING PATIENT

Few patients stress physicians as much as those who
are dying. This need not be. Even if little can be done
to change a fatal outcome, careful handling by the
physician and crucial others can help turn a patient's
death (whether expected or untimely) into a time of genuine
relief, satisfaction, and (even) growth. When time is so
limited, new realities and priorities emerge which must be
dealt with if life is to be concluded satisfactorily.

NORMAL RESPONSES IN THE DYING:

The news that one is dying produces a special kind of
grief reaction. A typical series of "stages" or psycho-

logical reactions to the threat of imminent death are seen
frequently (Kubler-Ross, 1970).

1st Stage - Shock and denial: Denial is the initial
    reaction of many patients to being told that they are
    dying - particularly severe in those "caught by
    surprise." They may refuse to believe the diagnosis,
    actively begin doctor-shopping, or be dazed and appear
    oblivious to the significance of the diagnosis. This
    may be fleeting, but some patients may never pass
    beyond this stage.
2nd Stage - Anger: A frustrated, hopeless, angry, bitter
    "Why me?" response often accompanies the realization
    of impending death. The anger is directed at the
    physicians (or family, God, fate, etc.) for the
    "unfairness" of this turn of events.
3rd Stage - Bargaining: The patient attempts to bargain
    with physicians or God for more time - promising good
    behavior, good intentions, etc; in exchange for: "a
    chance to see my boy be graduated from college," etc.
4th Stage - Depression: The patient despairs and begins to
    grieve. Be alert to suicide, particularly in the
    irritable, demanding, agitated depression.
5th Stage - Acceptance: The patient is quiet and resigned.
    He has little outside interests but seeks the presence
    of loved ones or a few close friends.

These stages are not necessarily stepwise and invariable.
Just as often the person will shift back and forth between
stages (eg, from denial to anger and then back to denial),
exhibit varying degrees of denial throughout, but gradually
become more detached. The younger the adult, the more
likely the stages are to be turbulent and the problems
severe.

    Specific psychiatric problems often occur and should
be identified and treated.

1. Depression is common but not "normal" and thus if a
    depression is not relieved by support and time, a
    Major Depression may have developed. Consider
    treatment with antidepressants.
2. Organic brain syndromes (usually waxing and waning)
    develop frequently and can be frightening to patients.
    Help them see the disorders as separate from
    themselves - as just another thing to be experienced.
3. Acute anxiety is common but usually temporary, particu-
    larly if treated with medication.
4. Communication failures between the patient and loved
    ones are very common and troublesome - often taking
    the form of a "tyranny of silence" or a lack of under-

standing on either one's part of the distress of the
other. These need to be dealt with directly.

TREATMENT:

Telling the Patient:

- Choose a quiet and private spot, be relaxed, sit down
  with the patient, and briefly reveal the diagnosis.
  Use the patient's response as an indicator of how much
  to tell.
- Patients need to know and need a chance to ask questions
  but, most of all, they need someone (usually the
  physician, but also spouse, pastor, etc) available -
  someone to help them grieve.
- Be truthful (but allow them to deny if they insist on it)
  and realistically hopeful ("We will begin treatment.
  Sometimes remissions occur. Etc."). Don't encourage
  false hopes but don't initially emphasize the fatal
  outcome.
- Strong negative reactions do occur. Sedation can be
  helpful temporarily.

Treating the Patient:

- Be supportive, empathic, warm, a good listener, hopeful
  (eg, about goals to be achieved before death), and
  available. Get to know the patient as a person -
  attention to exclusively medical matters is "dehuman-
  izing." Be tolerant of ups and downs. Recognize that
  the patient may become hostile towards you - help him
  work through it.

- Always take your lead from the patient. Some days some
  topics are too stressful. Other days they "have" to
  talk. Only force the issue if their denial, anxiety,
  or anger is seriously obstructing good care. Occasionally confrontation may be required.

- Make them comfortable. Treat pain aggressively -
  narcotics are OK. Attend fastidiously to basic
  physical needs. Make their room pleasant and
  cheerful. Hallucinogens (eg, LSD) have been used
  experimentally with success.

- Certain fears are common and need to be looked for and
  dealt with: eg, fear of pain, of physical dependency,
  of being isolated, of losing control (emotional and
  physical), of being helpless, of the unknown, of
  leaving loved ones to flounder (financially or
  emotionally.

- It is essential to help the patient "work through" the
  process of dying. Help him set new priorities and
  goals (eg, get his affairs in order). Help him
  resolve old problems and feel good about current
  relationships. Help him be responsible. Encourage
  him to consider not only how he will die but also how
  he will live the rest of his life.

- Do <u>not</u> insist that patients march through the "stages of
  dying" in a set order and on schedule.

- Allow the patient "terminal dependency" - it is OK finally
  to regress.

Treating the Family:

- Family members show many of the signs of grief. Like the
  patient, they also may be angry, hostile, or denying.
  They may need treatment - help <u>them</u> mourn.
- It is important to keep the family (ie, loved ones)
  involved. Help the patient die "with their blessing."
- It can be enormously beneficial (to the patient, to the
  family) if the patient can be supportive to the family
  members in their grieving.

Treating the Staff:

- Recognize that the physician, nurses, aides, etc. are all
  affected by death. Anxiety, intellectualization,
  avoidance, and grieving frequently occur among staff -
  don't let them impair care. Staff conferences to
  ventilate and explore these issues may help.

THE CHRONICALLY ILL PATIENT

Chronic illness is another form of stress which
entails grieving. Like the dying patient, these patients
may deny their illness, become angry and resentful,
regress, or become depressed. Common to all these
reactions is anxiety associated with a loss of health and
attractiveness, a loss of self-esteem, and the threat of
dependency or even death. Certain personality types are at
risk - eg, the narcissistic, the very independent.
Treatment principles useful with the grieving or dying
patient apply here as well.

REFERENCES

1. Atkinson RM, Henderson RG, Sparr LF, Deale S: Assessment of Viet Nam veterans for posttraumatic stress disorder in Veterans Administration disability claims. Am J Psychiat 139:1118, 1982.
2. Barry MJ: Therapeutic experience with patients referred for "prolonged grief reaction" - some second thoughts. Mayo Clin Proc 56:744, 1981.
3. Burgess AW, Holmstrom LL: Adaptive strategies and recovery from rape. Am J Psychiat 136:1278, 1979.
4. Clayton PJ: Mortality and morbidity in the first year of widowhood. Arch Gen Psychiat 30:747, 1974.
5. Falk N: Clinical management of rape. Hosp Physician 6:34, 1977.
6. Horowitz MJ, Wilner N, Kaltreider N, Alvarez W: Signs and symptoms of posttraumatic stress disorder. Arch Gen Psychiat 37:85, 1980.
7. Kubler-Ross E: On Death and Dying. London, Tavistock, 1970.
8. LaRoche C, Lalinec-Michand M, Engelsmann F, Fuller N, Copp M, Vasilevsky K: Grief reactions to perinatal death: an exploratory study. Psychosomatics 23:510, 1982.
9. Parkes CM: Bereavement: Studies of Grief in Adult Life. New York, International Univ Pr, 1972.
10. Sierles FS, Chen J-J, McFarland RE, Taylor MA: Posttraumatic stress disorder and concurrent psychiatric illness: a preliminary report. Am J Psychiat 140:1177, 1983.
11. Sparr L, Pankratz LD: Factitious posttraumatic stress disorder. Am J Psychiat 140:1016, 1983.
12. Stedeford A: Psychotherapy of the dying patient. Brit J Psychiat 135:7, 1979.
13. Wilkinson CB: Aftermath of a disaster: the collapse of the Hyatt Regency Hotel skywalks. Am J Psychiat 140:1134, 1983.
14. Zisook S, DeVaul RA: Grief, unresolved grief, and depression. Psychosomatics 24:247, 1983.
15. Zisook S, DeVaul RA, Clinck MA: Measuring symptoms of grief and bereavement. Am J Psychiat 139:1590, 1982.

Chapter 11

Conditions Which Mimic Physical Disease

It is essential to differentiate organic illness from psychogenic illness in patients complaining of physical symptoms. Patients with physical concerns in whom no medical illness can be found and/or who don't improve with treatment are common. These frustrating patients often exhaust one doctor after another and usually end up being labeled "hysterics" or "crocks." This occasionally angry response by the physician does a disservice to these patients since, although some may be consciously "faking it" (malingering), most patients have as yet undiagnosed organic conditions or have symptoms which are unconsciously and involuntarily produced.

There are several discrete involuntary psychiatric syndromes (somatoform disorders - see below) which mimic organic disease. These disorders have typical clinical presentations, family histories, recommended treatments, and likely prognoses.

Failure to identify an organic etiology for a physical symptom does not necessitate a diagnosis of a somatoform disorder or malingering - these are not diagnoses by exclusion but rather should be based on specific characteristics. Consider the following diagnoses in any patient with a poorly specified or uncertain medical conditon.

1. UNDETECTED PHYSICAL ILLNESS:

The possibility of an underlying, unrecognized illness must continue to be considered throughout the course of diagnosis and treatment, however long. Follow-up studies find 15-30% of conversion reaction diagnoses to represent misdiagnosed organic disease. Physical illness may produce symptoms which mimic a somatoform disorder or may pre-dispose susceptible patients to develop concurrent psychiatric conditions (it's not "either, or"). Some patients with subtle CNS disease are at risk for conversion symptoms so always carefully evaluate neurologically. The physical conditions commonly found (on follow-up) among these "false positive hysterics" include:

- CNS disease: Particularly epilepsy, MS, and post-concussion syndrome, but also CNS infections (eg, encephalitis), dementia, brain tumor, and cerebro-valcular disease.
- Degenerative disorders: Of musculo-skeletal and connective tissues; including SLE, polyarteritis nodosa, early rheumatoid arthritis, myasthenia gravis.
- Others: Syphilis, TB, hyper- and hypothyroidism, hyperparathyroidism, porphyria, hypoglycemia, duodenal and gallbladder disease, pancreatic disease, etc.

Be suspicious of any somatoform disorder which develops late in life. Psychological testing is of little help in differentiation - don't be misled by a "neurotic" picture on the MMPI into prematurely abandoning the search for a physical cause.

SOMATOFORM DISORDERS

2. CONVERSION DISORDER (Hysterical Neurosis, Conversion Type) (DSM-III p 244, 300.11):

A patient whose predominant problem is an obvious loss of function of some part of the nervous system which no identified organic pathology completely explains (conversion symptom) may have a conversion disorder. Conversion symptoms include:

Motor - paralysis, astasia-abasia, seizures, urinary retention, aphonia, globus hystericus ("lump in the throat" which prevents swallowing).
Sensory - paresthesia, anesthesia, anosmia, blindness, tunnel vision, deafness.
Other - unconsciousness, vomiting.

In addition, the particular symptom appears to serve one of two specific psychological purposes.

1. As primary gain, the symptom "buries" an unconscious mental conflict. An unacceptable, painful thought is repressed and the emotional energy is converted to a physical symptom. Usually the specific symptom "chosen" represents the conflict symbolically (eg, the negligent mother of a burned child develops anesthesia over the corresponding part of her body).

2. As secondary gain, the symptom gets the patient something he wants (eg, paralysis permits dependency on
   wife or justifies workman's compensation) or allows
   him to avoid something he doesn't want (eg, seizures
   prevent a court appearance).

Obvious as these relationships may be to the observer, the
patient is unaware of them (unconscious) and the patient
does not grasp their significance, even if they are
explained (lacks insight).

DIAGNOSIS:

   In the apparent absence of organic pathology, it is
necessary to identify features in addition to a presumed
conversion symptom before making the diagnosis. Realize
also that as many as 25% of patients with conversion
disorders have associated organic pathology (eg, epilepsy
in a patient with pseudoseizures) so also investigate
symptoms only partially explained by the physical abnormalities. Features associated with conversion disorders
include:

- The symptom occurs abruptly and frequently follows an
  acute stress.
- There is often a past history of the same or a different
  conversion symptom.
- The disorder usually is seen first during adolescence or
  in the patient's 20's and in a person predisposed by a
  dependent, histrionic, antisocial, or passive-
  aggressive personality disorder.
- The patients often have associated moderate anxiety and
  depression.
- The purpose the symptom serves is occasionally quickly
  apparent.
- The patients are frequently immature, shallow, and
  demanding although they tend to cooperate with
  examinations. They tend to have lower intelligence,
  limited insight, and lower socioeconomic status.
- Indifference to the symptom may be found (la belle
  indifference).

   The individual neurologic symptoms may have some
characteristics which distinguish them from those of an
organic etiology. In general, they tend to be variable,
atypical, and inconsistent with anatomy.

Conversion Seizures: Seizures are often atypical and
   bizarre (patient may laugh or cry throughout seizure).
   Only infrequently is there incontinence, cyanosis,
   physical self-harm, tongue biting, or complete loss of

consciousness during the seizure. Good muscle tone is
preserved during the, typically brief, postictal stage
(arm dropped onto face may land lightly or miss the
face altogether). The onset is usually dramatic and
seizures rarely occur when the patient is alone. Sit
patient quickly upright - seizures often stop.

Conversion Unconsciousness: The loss of consciousness is
usually light and incomplete with the patient showing
some awareness of environmental events, particularly
when he feels unobserved. VS and reflexes are normal
and the patient usually responds to painful stimuli.
The eyes are held tightly shut and some movements may
be purposive (eg, move to keep from falling from exam
table).

Conversion Paralysis: The paralysis is often variable -
even during one exam. Paralysis of one limb or part
of a limb, or hemiparesis are most common but the
specific involvement is often inconsistent with
anatomy and the related changes (eg, tone, etc) are
atypical. DTR changes are variable and pathological
reflexes (eg, Babinski) are not present. The paralyzed limbs often show little resistance to passive
movement but resist the pull of gravity. If there is
resistance to forced movement, it tends to give way
abruptly (vs gradually as in organic conditions).
There may be movement when startled by a painful
stimulus. Palpate the antagonists - they often con-
tract to simulate agonist weakness. There are usually
associated conversion sensory changes.

Astasia-abasia: This exaggerated and bizarre conversion
ataxia varies from moment to moment. The patient
falls toward walls and people, rarely falls to the
floor, and rarely hurts himself in spite of a dramatic
presentation.

Conversion Sensory Changes: These are often dramatic,
sometimes vague, and usually inconsistent with anatomy
(eg, "stocking and glove" anesthesia, loss of all
senses on one side or below a certain level on a limb,
loss which stops exactly at midline. Careful testing
differentiates most cases.

Conversion Blindness: Visual disturbances are usually
blurring, double vision, or tunnel loss but may be
total blindness. Response to a bright light (check
with EEG) and avoidance of threatening objects are
often inconsistent with the degree of presumed visual
loss.

When the diagnosis is in doubt, a single dose of IV sodium amobarbital (Amytal) often temporarily removes the conversion symptom, thus clarifying the diagnosis. Slowly give a 10% solution intravenously (1 ml/min - maximum of 500 mg). When the patient's words begin to slur, stop administration and observe for disappearance of symptom.

DIFFERENTIAL DIAGNOSIS:

- Carefully rule out physical illness.
- Some patients with conversion symptoms require a primary diagnosis of major depression or schizophrenia.
- Two somatoform disorders (see below) have features in common with conversion disorders - somatization disorder and psychogenic pain disorder.
- Differentiation from malingering is difficult (see below).

TREATMENT:

Some patients have a short course and are "spontaneous cures," a few may be chronic (eg, some paralyzed patients actually develop contractures), but most improve over weeks or months. A physical process is later identified in a significant minority (25%).

It is uncertain what treatment is best. Long-term psychoanalysis appears to effect real change in a few but is not for the majority of patients. Use minor tranquilizers if anxiety predominates. Behavior modification has had mixed success.

Crucial to any therapy is the formation of a supportive therapeutic alliance, but these patients are generally resistant to treatment. Direct confrontation about the "hysterical" nature of the symptom rarely works - the patient usually withdraws. Help the patient ventilate. Help the patient explore areas of stress in her life but relate that to symptoms only after an alliance has been formed. Gradually identify the symbolic nature of the symptoms, if present.

Work with the family. Help restructure the patient's environment to remove the secondary gain, if possible. Educate other involved medical personnel about the disorder - help them avoid countertherapeutic hostility.

3. SOMATIZATION DISORDER (Hysteria, Briquet's Syndrome) (DSM-III p 241, 300.81):

This syndrome has been delineated in the last few years and may or may not be coequal to the traditional diagnosis of hysteria. The patients have numerous vague and dramatic physical symptoms (usually presented in a dramatic way) which typically involve several organ systems.

- Conversion symptoms of all types
- Vague and ill-defined pains
- Menstrual problems; inhibited orgasm
- GI, GU, and cardiopulmonary difficulties
- Poorly characterized altered states of consciousness

The symptoms wax and wane but usually are presented forcefully by the patient who insists on examination and treatment. These patients often receive multiple operations and are at risk for iatrogenically induced drug addiction.

Analytically oriented researchers argue that symptoms are produced when forbidden impulses are repressed and the emotional energy associated with those drives is converted (conversion) into a physical symptom. Although definitive information remains incomplete, features currently associated with Briquet's Syndrome include:

- A chronic condition beginning in adolescence or during the 20's.
- Primarily in women; 1% of all women.
- Anxiety, irritability, and depression common; frequent suicide attempts (but few successful).
- Patients usually of lower intelligence and lower socio-economic groups.
- Frequent interpersonal and marital problems.
- Patients often have a previous or concurrent history of antisocial behavior and a poor school history.
- Patients may have histrionic personality disorder or antisocial personality disorder.
- First-degree female relatives have a 20% incidence of somatization disorder. First-degree male relatives have increased prevalence of alcoholism and anti-social personality disorder.

Somatization disorder is difficult to distinguish from malingering and occasionally there are elements of both present. It is essential to rule out inconstant and confusing medical syndromes (eg, SLE, acute intermittent porphyria, temporal lobe epilepsy, MS, hyperparathyroidism) although most can be differentiated from the full Briquet's Syndrome (reliable diagnostic screening tests are avialable - Reveley, 1977). Follow-up studies find few cases of undiagnosed organic illness (unlike conversion disorder). Rule out somatization in schizophrenia and depression.

TREATMENT:

Treatment success is limited. Focus usually should be placed on management rather than cure. Develop a therapeutic alliance by being sympathetic and interested in the patient and her health but don't make that your exclusive focus. Gradually encourage an examination of the patient's general life problems and coping styles. Help the patient develop mature social, occupational, and intimate interpersonal skills. Treat depression and anxiety with medication, if indicated, but recognize the risk for addiction.

4. <u>PSYCHOGENIC PAIN DISORDER</u> (DSM-III p 247, 307.80):

These patients (often women) experience pain for which no cause can be found. It appears suddenly, usually following a stress, and may disappear in days or last years. This condition is very similar to conversion disorder and the patients may differ only by experiencing pain rather than neurological deficit as the predominant symptom (Bishop, 1979). Treatments are also similar.

5. <u>HYPOCHONDRIASIS</u> (Hypochondriacal Neurosis) (DSM-III p 249, 300.70):

Although many people may mentally expand a minor symptom into a major physical illness (particularly during times of stress), they rarely become preoccupied with it and can easily be dissuaded when examination and laboratory tests are normal. The hypochondriac, on the other hand, is convinced he is ill, angrily rejects evidence to the contrary, insists on further tests and treatments, and feverishly doctor shops. The patient appears pleased only if assured he is sick and he eagerly seeks additional medical attention. This common chronic condition begins in adolescence or middle age, is common among the elderly, and is resistant to therapy. The patient rarely sees a psychiatrist but rather drifts from internist to surgeon to neurologist etc.

The patient is hyperalert to symptoms and presents them in great detail during the history. He usually has some specific idea of "what the trouble is" and merely may want the physician to concur. Physicians frequently become angry and rejecting toward the patient which leads to further "shopping around." In severe cases, the patient becomes an invalid.

Many of these patients display anxiety or depression. Hypochondriacal features occur frequently in serious psychiatric conditions like schizophrenia, major depression, dysthymic disorder, and organic brain syndromes. Rule out other somatoform disorders, chronic factitious disorder, and malingering.

Treatment is unpromising. Symptoms may disappear if an associated depression or psychosis is successfully treated. Don't expect a "cure" but rather work with the patient to help control his symptoms. "Assure" the patient that the problem is persistent but not debilitating or fatal. See the patient frequently for short periods of time. Assure him that you will be available if needed but schedule regular appointments (to be kept whether or not he is feeling ill). Consider giving a mild medication (eg, antihistamine, vitamin) which can be a focus of attention during appointments and will be evidence that he is taken seriously. This form of palliation can restore the patient to functional health more readily than any definitive medical treatment.

SIMULATION OF PHYSICAL SYMPTOMS

Two categories of patients voluntarily mimic physical symptoms:

6. MALINGERING (DSM-III p 331, V65.20):

These people knowingly fake symptoms for some obvious gain. They may be trying to get drugs, avoid the law, get a bed for the night, etc. In spite of their physical complaints, they tend to be evasive and uncooperative during evaluation and therapy, and they avoid medical procedures. When exposed, they may angrily give up their symptoms and sign out AMA. Antisocial personality disorder and drug abuse are common associated conditions.

7. CHRONIC FACTITIOUS DISORDER WITH PHYSICAL SYMPTOMS (Munchausen Syndrome) (DSM-III p 288, 301.51):

These patients also knowingly fake symptoms but do so for unconscious psychological reasons that become evident after a thorough psychiatric evaluation. They usually prefer the sick role and move from hospital to hospital in what is a chronic life pattern. They are usually loners with an early childhood background of trauma and deprivation. They are unable to establish close interpersonal relationships and generally have severe personality disorders. Unlike many malingerers, they follow through with medical procedures and are at risk for drug addiction and for the complications of multiple operations.

Both groups of patients can be difficult to distinguish from the somatoform disorders and from organic illness yet careful and repeated examinations will usually uncover their deceptions. The most common presentations include:

- Abdominal pain: May have an abdomen "like a railroad yard."
- Heart: Complains of pain. May induce arrhythmias with digitalis or produce tachycardia with amphetamines or thyroid.
- Bleeding: Patient may take anticoagulants or add blood from a scratch to lab samples.
- Neurological: Weakness, seizures, unconsciousness - difficult to differentiate from conversion symptoms.
- Fever: Produced by manipulating the thermometer (eg, hot coffee in the mouth).
- Skin: Look for lesions in a linear pattern in areas the patient can reach.

Although they both produce symptoms consciously, they should be dealt with differently. The malingerer should be handled formally (and often legally). The patient with a factitious disorder should be treated sympathetically and every effort made to convince him to enter psychotherapy (difficult). Unlike the malingerer, these patients are unable to control their self-destructive behavior and this should be tactfully pointed out to them.

REFERENCES

1. Adler G: The physician and the hypochondriacal patient. NEJM 304:1394, 1981.
2. Barsky AJ, Klerman GL: Overview: hypochondriasis, bodily complaints, and somatic styles. Am J Psychiat 140:273, 1983.
3. Bishop ER, Torch EM: Dividing "hysteria": a preliminary investigation of conversion disorder and psychalgia. J Nerv Ment Dis 167:348, 1979.
4. Cohen LM: A current perspective of pseudocyesis. Am J Psychiat 139:1140, 1982.
5. Dejong RN: The Neurologic Examination, ed 4. Hagerstown, Harper & Row, 1979.
6. Drossman DA: Patients with psychogenic abdominal pain: six years observation in the medical setting. Am J Psychiat 139:1549, 1982.
7. Ford CV: The Somatizing Disorders. New York, Elsevier Biomedical, 1983.
8. Goodwin DW, Guze SB: Psychiatric Diagnosis, ed 2. New York, Oxford Univ Pr, 1979.

9. Guberman A: Psychogenic pseudoseizures in non-epileptic
    patients. Can J Psychiat 27:401, 1982.
10. Henderson LM, Bell BA, Miller JD: A neurosurgical
    munchausen tale. J Neur Neursurg Psychiat 46:437, 1983.
11. Kellner R: Prognosis of treated hypochondriasis. Acta
    Psychiatr Scand 67:69, 1983.
12. Kellner R: Psychotherapeutic strategies in hypochondri-
    asis: a clinical study. Am J Psychotherapy 36:146,
    1982.
13. Reveley MA, Woodruff RA, Robins LN, Taibleson M,
    Reich T, Helzer J: Evaluation of a screening interview
    for Briquet Syndrome (Hysteria) by the study of
    medically ill women. Arch Gen Psychiat 34:145, 1977.
14. Riley TL, Roy A: Pseudoseizures. Baltimore, Williams &
    Wilkins, 1982.
15. Weintraub MI: Hysterical Conversion Reactions. New
    York, SP Med & Scient Bks, 1983.

Chapter 12

Psychosomatic Disorders

A psychosomatic disorder is a physical disease partially caused or exacerbated by psychological factors (PSYCHOLOGICAL FACTORS AFFECTING PHYSICAL CONDITIONS, DSM-III p 303, 316.00). This classification applies only to those conditions in which psychological influence is of major significance - but be aware that any physical disease may be modified by psychological stress. The term "psychosomatic" does not refer to:

1. A physical symptom or clinical presentation caused by psychological factors for which there is no organic basis (eg, conversion disorder, psychogenic pain disorder, somatization disorder).
2. A patient with numerous physical complaints but without organic pathology (eg, somatization disorder, hypochondriasis, malingering).
3. Physical complaints related to habit disorders - eg, dyspnea due to excessive smoking.

MECHANISMS OF DISEASE PRODUCTION:

There are many specific diseases which are influenced greatly by the "psyche" (see below) but, although much studied, the mechanisms by which the brain produces such organic pathology are unclear.

Psychological mechanisms:

"Stress," either internal or external, is required but is much more likely to cause disease if:

1. The stress is severe (eg, death of a loved one, divorce or separation, major illness or injury, financial crisis, incarceration). Holmes and Rahe (1967) developed a ranked scale of stressful life events (rated by life change units - LCU) and found a close correlation between an event's stress (in LCUs) and

the patient's likelihood of developing a physical illness.
2. The stress is chronic.
3. The patient perceives the stress as stressful.
4. The patient has an increased level of general instability - eg, difficult job, troubled marriage, urban dweller, socially disrupted environment, etc.

It was once thought (F. Dunbar) that _specific_ superficial personality traits produced specific organic diseases (eg, that there is a "coronary personality," an "ulcer personality," etc). It was also held (F. Alexander) that _specific_ deep and unconscious, unresolved neurotic conflicts caused specific physical disorders. Currently, the only specificity that is generally accepted associates the "Type A" personality (ie, sense of time urgency, impatience, aggressiveness, upward striving, competitiveness, tendency to anger when frustrated) with coronary artery disease (Friedman and Rosenman, 1971).

More generally accepted are _nonspecific_ hypotheses which link a wide variety of stresses to the development of disease in an individual placed at risk by one or more of the following:

1. A genetic susceptibility.
2. A degree of chronic debilitation, a current illness, or an "organ vulnerability."
3. A tendency to react to stress with anger, resentment, frustration, anxiety, or depression.
4. A "psychological susceptibility" (eg, patient is pessimistic and "expects the worst" vs being optimistic and actively working to overcome stress).
5. An "alexithymic" personality - eg, a person who is in poor contact with his emotions and has an impoverished fantasy life.

Physiological mechanisms:

These mechanisms are poorly understood and only the broad outline can be sketched. Stress is perceived cognitively (by the cerebral cortex) but, once recognized, is mediated primarily by the limbic system which, under chronic stress, chronically stimulates the hypothalamus and the vegetative centers in the brain stem. This stimulation produces a direct effect on the various organs by:

1. Activation of the autonomic nervous system (sympathetic and adrenal medulla; parasympathetic).
2. Involvement of the neuroendocrine system - ie, releasing hormones from the hypothalamus travel

through the pituitary portal system to the anterior
pituitary where they cause the release of the
trophic hormones (eg, ACTH, TSH, GH, FSH) which
either act directly or release other hormones from
the endocrine glands (eg, cortisol, thyroxin,
epinephrine, NE, sex hormones). These produce a
variety of changes in structures throughout the
body. Hans Selye (1976) emphasized the central
role of cortisol as a primary mediator of the
body's stress response (general adaptation syndrome
- GAS) - if cortisol is released too chronically,
various organs are damaged, producing psychosomatic
diseases.

The details have yet to be worked out - there remain more
questions than answers. The recently identified hormones,
endorphins, may play a major role in stress response
regulation. Central to all of these physiological systems
is the concept of homeostasis - psychosomatic diseases
occur when the body's "natural balance" is upset,
particularly if it is chronically upset.

Although psychosomatic medicine has been concerned
primarily with those diseases felt to be "psychosomatic,"
recently the concept has been broadened to include (or
overlap with) the new field of Behavioral Medicine. The
essence of behavioral medicine (Pomerleau and Brady, 1979)
is the application of behavior modification techniques
derived from learning theory to various medical problems -
eg, chronic pain, hypertension and other psychosomatic
diseases, habit disorders, etc. Techniques used include
behavioral self-management methods, biofeedback, hypnosis,
and various relaxation procedures.

SPECIFIC PSYCHOSOMATIC DISORDERS:

Although (1) stress can increase the susceptibility to
any disease and (2) most diseases are currently viewed as
multifactorially determined, those that most clearly have a
major psychosomatic contribution include the following
disorders.

CARDIOVASCULAR:

Coronary artery disease: More common in "Type A"
personalities. These patients have increased serum
cholesterol, low-density lipoproteins, and tri-
glycerides; also increased urinary 17-ketosteroids,
17-hydroxycorticosteroids, and NE. Sudden death by MI
is increased in patients experiencing a severe recent
loss (1st 6 months).

Hypertension: Chronic psychosocial stress probably plays
a role in its development in genetically predisposed
patients. Mechanism is uncertain but may not be
related to the brief hypertension that occurs during
periods of acute stress. May occur more frequently in
Type A people and in compulsive people who "store
resentment" and who handle angry feelings poorly.
Treat first with antihypertensives. Relaxation
therapy (eg, progressive relaxation, meditation,
hypnosis) is an effective adjunct to drugs - biofeedback may also help.

Arrhythmias: Palpitation, sinus tachycardia, and
worsening of pre-existing arrhythmias may all be
produced by stress - probably via a sympathetic-
parasympathetic imbalance.

Hypotension (fainting): Produced by fear - probably due
to peripheral vasodilation and a decreased ventricular
filling.

Congestive heart failure: Frequently develops following
periods of stress. Anxiety tends to exacerbate the
condition.

Raynaud's Disease: Can often be treated effectively with
progressive relaxation or biofeedback.

Migraine: Attacks are often precipitated by stress.
Treatment should include medication and biofeedback.
Consider relaxation and psychotherapy also.

RESPIRATORY:

Bronchial Asthma: Occurs in people with a genetic
predisposition - made worse by acute and chronic
stress. These patients are at risk for developing
neurotic emotional reactions secondary to the
respiratory disorder. There is good evidence that a
wide variety of problem-solving and stress-reducing
techniques (eg, psychotherapy, family therapy,
systematic desensitization, hypnosis, etc) are
effective at preventing attacks in many asthmatics and
should be used in conjunction with medication (Creer,
1980).

Hay fever: Patients have an increased sensitivity to
their allergens when stressed but may also develop
characteristic symptoms when no allergens can be
identified.

Tuberculosis: Chronic stress often precedes development
of the disease.

Hyperventilation syndrome: A common ER presentation (see
chapter 8). Differentiate from panic disorder.

GASTROINTESTINAL:

Peptic Ulcer: Stress contributes to ulcer development,
    probably through its influence on the hypothalamic-
    pituitary-adrenal axis. The chronically frustrated
    and angry patient with increased gastric HCL
    (hypersecretor) is at risk. Help the patient develop
    more stress-free life patterns. Relaxation therapy
    may be of value.
Ulcerative Colitis: Stressful emotional factors often
    precede disease development and can induce a relapse
    but the mechanism is unclear. Non-confrontive,
    supportive psychotherapy is indicated to help the
    patient adapt better to stress and to his illness and
    to help him deal with the frequently associated
    anxiety and depression, but psychiatric care alone
    will not prevent relapses. Other intestinal
    conditions which are markedly influenced by psycho-
    social stress include regional enteritis (Crohn's
    Disease) and irritable bowel syndrome.
Obesity: Genetic and psychological factors interact.
    Improper conditioning around food habits, an over-
    valuation of food, and a negative body image (eg,
    "fatso") are central. "Binge eaters" are particularly
    susceptible to stress. Supportive psychotherapy may
    be of some value but behavior modification is most
    useful (Howard, 1975). Long-term success is limited -
    initial weight loss is frequent but relapses are very
    common. A change in life-style appears essential.
ANOREXIA NERVOSA (DSM-III p 67, 307.10): This disorder
    of profound weight loss without loss of appetite
    usually develops in adolescence (F:M = 10:1),
    continues through the early 20's, and may end in death
    by starvation (5-10%). It is increasingly common in
    upper middle class females.
        These patients have a disturbed body image (feel
    fat in spite of dramatic visual evidence to the
    contrary) and are preoccupied with losing weight.
    They diet, exercise, and dangerously abuse diuretics
    and laxatives, even while family members and profes-
    sionals attempt to stop them. Many anorexics (50% at
    some time during their course) also binge eat.
        A related condition, BULIMIA (DSM-III p 69,
    307.51), is a chronic disorder characterized primarily
    by episodic eating binges in adolescent or early adult
    females (F:M = 10-20:1) of normal weight who follow
    the gorging by self-induced vomiting or by inducing
    diarrhea with laxatives. These individuals are weight
    conscious and markedly depressed by their uncontrolled
    eating. Self-deprecation and suicidal ruminations are
    common. Endocrinological, family history, and treat-

ment findings are similar to those of anorexics and many patients slip back and forth between the two conditions over time.

Anorexics often have hormone imbalances (eg, amenorrhea), numerous signs of starvation (eg, edema, bradycardia, and hypothermia), and associated features like ritual behavior (eg, hand-washing). The etiology is uncertain. The families frequently have disturbed interpersonal patterns and an increased incidence of eating and affective disorders. Be certain to rule out a primary affective or schizophrenic disorder.

Treatment should involve hospitalization for severe cases, individual and family therapy, and behavior modification. Some patients (particularly bulimics) improve with antidepressants, while a few require antipsychotics. In its early stages this condition is frequently overlooked yet treatment can be life-saving. Develop a high index of suspicion in thin, young females.

MUSCULOSKELETAL:

Rheumatoid Arthritis: Symptoms frequently worsen following emotional stress. Stress may be acting as an immunosuppressant. Depression is common in these patients. Psychotherapy is of little value in altering the course of the disease.

Tension headaches: Caused by chronic muscular tension. Treat with mild analgesics and EMG feedback from the frontalis muscles or with relaxation techniques (often coupled with vigorous activity).

Spasmodic torticollis: Exacerbated by stress. EMG biofeedback may be useful.

Low back pain: Treat multimodally.

ENDOCRINE:

Conditions which are exacerbated by stress include hyperthyroidism and diabetes mellitus. Acute and chronic stress may precipitate a thyroid crisis in genetically predisposed patients. Ketosis may be produced and maintained by stress in diabetics. Patients with either condition should receive psychotherapy if they have adopted self-destructive life habits and if they experience frequent relapses.

GENITOURINARY:

Most gynecological disorders reflect primarily an endocrine imbalance but many of these conditions also can be influenced significantly by psychosocial stress.

Psychosomatic influences are most evident for: menstrual disorders (premenstrual tension, amenorrhea, oligomenorrhea), dyspareunia, frigidity, pseudocyesis, premature ejaculation, and impotence. Spontaneous abortion can be produced by major stress.

CHRONIC PAIN:

Chronic pain patients are common. The sources of their pain may or may not be identifiable. They often have been thoroughly evaluated medically, have experienced several unsuccessful surgical or medical procedures, and may or may not be currently iatrogenically addicted to analgesics (be wary of requests for Demerol, Percodan, Codeine, Darvon, Talwin, Valium, etc). Nothing has helped and the patients show evidence of depression, hopelessness, chronic anxiety, insomnia, chronic anger, interpersonal withdrawal, and/or somatic preoccupation. Their lives may be totally dominated by the pain.

Be certain that you are not dealing with conditions which mimic or complicate chronic pain (see chapter 11):

1. Unrecognized, treatable organic pathology
2. Primary depression, anxiety disorder, or psychosis
3. Unrecognized, early OBS
4. Drug addiction
5. Conversion disorder
6. Somatization disorder
7. Psychogenic pain disorder
8. Hypochondriasis
9. Histrionic personality disorder
10. Malingering
11. Compensation factors

Always treat the chronic pain patient globally. Do not become overly concerned about whether the pain is "real" or "psychological" - it invariably will have elements of both and treatments often will be similar. Use whatever medical and surgical means are of value but do not stop there. Always explore and apply the multiplicity of psychological treatments that are available.

- First, detoxify the patient, if necessary.
- Take the patient and his pain seriously. Be interested, sympathetic, and hopeful. Be a continuing presence - see the patient regularly and do not abandon him.
- Help the patient identify and accept reasonable expect- ations. Encourage him to continue functioning - avoid hospitalization.

- Recognize that chronic administration of analgesics has limited usefulness and great risks yet can be done therapeutically. Attempt to use no drugs or non-addicting drugs (eg, antidepressants, major tranquilizers, antihistamines). Codeine is the preferable narcotic.
- Have the patient keep a pain diary. Work with the patient over time to help him determine what variables improve or worsen the pain.
- Consider the variety of psychological techniques available - eg, hypnosis, biofeedback, relaxation therapy, etc. Encourage the patient to discover that he is "in control of his own pain." Use these methods within the context of a good therapeutic alliance. Consider family and group therapy. Help others in the patient's environment become more appropriately responsive to his pain.
- Consider some physical procedures - eg, nerve block, dorsal column stimulators, acupuncture, rhizotomy, etc. Avoid surgery if possible.
- Recognize that not all patients will improve markedly.

OTHER:

Skin: A wide variety of psychosocial stressors can exacerbate certain skin conditions, including psoriasis, chronic urticaria, pruritis, neuro-dermatitis (eczema), and trichotillomania. There is good research to suggest that warts (a contagious disease) responds to hypnosis (Surman et al, 1973).

Malignant disease: Psychological stressors appear to influence the development and course of a malignancy. This may be related to the effect of stress on the immune system. Much work remains to be done, yet there is some suggestion that psychological treatments (eg, hypnosis) may play a future role in cancer treatment.

Hematological: Stress may aid clotting among hemophiliacs. Changes in levels of various blood elements may occur in normals under acute stress.

Accident proneness: Some people are chronically at risk for accidental trauma due to psychological character-istics (eg, impulsive, anxious, hostile).

Seizures: Emotional stress can trigger seizures (both neurogenic and conversion). Psychotherapy and stress management is effective in helping to control seizure disorders, particularly in patients with partial seizures.

REFERENCES

1. Adams HE, Feuerstein M, Fowler JL: Migraine headache:

review of parameters, etiology, and intervention. Psychological Bulletin 87:217, 1980.

2. Alexander F, French T: Psychosomatic Specificity, Vol I. Chicago, Univ Chicago Pr, 1968.

3. Creer TL: Self-management behavioral strategies for asthamtics. Behavioral Med 7:14, March, 1980.

4. Friedman M, Rosenman RH: Type A behavior pattern: its association with coronary heart disease. Am Clin Res 3:300, 1971.

5. Haggerty JJ: The psychosomatic family: an overview. Psychosomatics 24:615, 1983.

6. Halmi KA: Anorexia nervosa and bulimia. Psychosomatics 24:111, 1983.

7. Holmes TH, Rahe RH: The social readjustment rating scale. J Psychosom Res 11:213, 1967.

8. Hudson JI, Pope HG, Jonas JM, Yurgelun-Todd D: Family history study of anorexia nervosa and bulimia. Brit J Psychiat 142:133, 1983.

9. Johnson C, Berndt DJ: Preliminary investigation of bulimia and life adjustment. Am J Psychiat 140:774, 1983.

10. Latimer PR: Irritable bowel syndrome. Psychosomatics 24:205, 1983.

11. Latimer PR: External contingency management for chronic pain: critical review of the evidence. Am J Psychiat 139:1308, 1982.

12. Lesser IM, Lesser BZ: Alexithymia: examining the development of a psychological concept. Am J Psychiat 140:1305, 1983.

13. Pomerleau OF, Brady JP: Behavioral Medicine: Theory and Practice. Baltimore, Williams & Wilkins Co, 1979.

14. Pope HG, Hudson JI, Jonas JM: Antidepressant treatment of bulimia: preliminary experience and practical recommendations. J Clin Psychopharm 3:274, 1983.

15. Reich J, Tupin JP, Abramowitz SI: Psychiatric diagnosis of chronic pain patients. Am J Psychiat 140:1495, 1983.

16. Selye H: The Stress of Life, 2nd ed. New York, McGraw-Hill Book Co, 1976.

17. Stunkard AJ: The current status of treatment for obesity in adults. Psychiat Ann 13:862, 1983.

18. Surman OS, Gottlieb SK, Hackett TP, Silverberg, EL: Hypnosis in the treatment of warts. Arch Gen Psychiat 28:439, 1973.

19. Taylor CB, Fortmann SP: Essential hypertension. Psychosomatics 24:433, 1983.

20. Webb WL: Chronic pain. Psychosomatics 24:1053, 1983.

Chapter 13

Psychiatric Symptoms of Nonpsychiatric Medication

Many medical patients develop psychiatric symptoms due to treatment with medical drugs - (1) as a common side effect, (2) as an idiosyncratic response, (3) from administration of toxic amounts, or (4) as the result of an untoward combination of drugs. Unrecognized, the responsible medications might be continued. Likely offenders include:

ANTICONVULSANTS:

Diphenylhydantoin, phenacemide: Irritability, emotional lability, confusion, and occasionally hallucinations and psychotic thinking - at times with normal blood levels. Symptoms occur more frequently in patients who also demonstrate tremor and ataxia.

Phenobarbital: Normal blood levels occasionally may produce irritability and/or confusion in the elderly while excessive dosage will produce oversedation. Symptoms of withdrawal may occur if phenobarbital is stopped abruptly.

ANTI-INFLAMMATORY AGENTS:

Phenylbutazone (Butazolidin): Anxiety, nervousness, emotional lability.

Indomethacin (Indocin): Dizziness, disorientation, and confusion; also occasionally depression, hallucinations, and psychosis.

Salicylates: Can produce elation and euphoria grading into confusion and depression in high doses.

HORMONES:

Exogenous thyroid: Excess can result in symptoms varying
from restlessness and anxiety to a psychosis mimicking
mania or acute schizophrenia. Inadequately treated
patients may display symptoms of hypothyroidism; eg,
fatigue, depression, psychosis (myxedema madness).

Adrenal corticosteroids (eg, cortisone, dexamethasone,
prednisone): In addition to physical complications,
excessive or chronic use can produce widely varying
affective syndromes (eg, euphoria and hypomania,
fatigue and depression) and/or degrees of a toxic
psychosis. Steroid withdrawal can produce complaints
of weakness and fatigue - suspect pseudotumor cerebri
if coupled with headache, vomiting, and confusion.

Estrogens: Restlessness, a sense of well-being, euphoria.

Progesterones: May produce fatigue, irritability,
tearfulness, and depression when given either alone or
in combination as oral contraceptives (2-30% of
patients).

Androgens: Restlessness, agitation, aggressiveness,
euphoria.

ANTICHOLINERGICS:

An anticholinergic psychosis (see chapter 23) can be
caused by a variety of medical drugs as can milder
peripheral (dry mouth, hypotension) and central (lability,
distractibility, restlessness) side effects.

Antihistamines: eg, Benadryl, Phenergan, Teldrin,
Ornade, Dramamine.

Antispasmodics: eg, Banthine.

Ophthalmic drops: eg, atropine, homatropine,
cyclopentolate.

Antiparkinsonian drugs: eg, Cogentin, Artane, Tremin,
Kemadrin, Akineton.

Others: Compoz, Excedrin PM, Sleep-Eze, Sominex and
others containing scopolamine.

Treat psychosis with physostigmine 1-2 mg, IM or
slowly IV; repeat in 20 minutes if needed.

ANTIHYPERTENSIVES:

Rauwolfia Alkaloids (reserpine): Can cause nightmares,
confusion, and profound depression in susceptible
patients taking normal doses.

Diuretics (thiazides, furosimide, ethacrynic acid):
Fatigue and mild depression.

Methyldopa (Aldomet): Persistent lassitude; verbal memory
impairment; depression with obtundation and confusion
(on normal dosage).
Guanethidine (Ismelin): mild depression.
Clonidine: sedation, depression; antagonized by tricyclic
antidepressants.

CARDIAC DRUGS:

Digitalis and the cardiac glycosides: Fatigue, apathy,
depression, and/or toxic delirium - particularly in
the elderly.
Propranolol (Inderal): Fatigue, insomnia, nightmares,
verbal memory impairment, and depression; rarely
confusion and a toxic psychosis.
Antiarrhythmics (quinidine, procainamide, lidocaine):
Grades of confusion and mild to major delirium;
occasionally depression.

SYMPATHOMIMETICS:

Both catecholamine and noncatecholamine stimulants may
produce restlessness, anxiety, fear and panic, weakness,
dizziness, irritability, and insomnia in recommended
dosages.

BROMIDE:

Acute intoxication is rare - bromide is too irritating
to allow ingestion of large doses. Symptoms of chronic
intoxication (weeks, months) (bromism) range from mild
disorientation to full toxic psychosis. Look for
"classic" acneiform rash of face and hair roots (30% of
patients) in persons using some over-the-counter
sedatives (eg, Bromo-Seltzer).

L-DOPA:

The depression and apathy of Parkinson's disease may
be relieved but anxiety and agitation are produced
frequently. 15% of patients develop more serious
psychiatric problems including an acute organic brain
syndrome with confusion or frank delirium, hypomania,
acute psychosis, or major depression. Often hard to
differentiate from the progression of the disease.

HYPOGLYCEMICS (insulin, tolbutamide, phenformin):

Symptoms of hypoglycemia - restlessness, anxiety,
disorientation.

ANTIBIOTICS and related drugs:

Tetracyclines: Can produce emotional lability, depression, and confusion - from vitamin deficiencies secondary to alteration of colonic bacteria.
Nalidixic acid and nitrofurantoin: Lethargy; rarely confusion.
Isoniazid (INH): Euphoria, transient memory loss, agitation, psychotic reaction, paranoia, catatonic-like syndrome.
Cycloserine: Lethargy and confusion, agitation, severe depression, psychosis, paranoid reactions.

ANTINEOPLASTICS:

Acute organic brain syndromes and depression can be produced by a variety of these agents - either by a direct CNS effect or due to involvement of other systems (eg, anemia).

REFERENCES

1. Bernstein JG: Medical-psychiatric drug interactions, in Hackett TP, Cassem NH: Handbook of General Hospital Psychiatry. St. Louis, CV Mosby Co, 1978.
2. Carpenter WT, Gruen PH: Cortisol's effects on human mental functioning. J Clin Psychopharm 2:91, 1982.
3. David K: Psychological effects of non-psychiatric drugs, in Barchas J: Psychopharmacology: From Theory to Practice. New York, Oxford Univ Pr, 1977.
4. Hall RC: Psychiatric Presentations of Medical Illness. New York, SP Medical & Scientific Books, 1980.
5. Hall RC, Popkin MK, Stickney SK, Gardner ER: Presentation of the steroid psychoses. J Nerv Ment Dis 167:229, 1979.
6. Shader RI: Psychiatric Complication of Medical Drugs. New York, Raven Pr, 1972.
7. Solomon S, Hotchkiss E, Saravay SM, Bayer C, Ramsey P, Blum RS: Impairment of memory function by antihypertensive medication. Arch Gen Psychiat 40:1109, 1983.
8. Walker S: Psychiatric Signs and Symptoms Due to Medical Problems. Springfield, Thomas Pub, 1967.

Chapter 14

Psychiatric Presentations of Medical Disease

Physical and psychiatric illnesses are closely interwoven. Both medical and psychiatric physicians should appreciate this interrelationship.

- 60% of patients needing mental health care are being treated by medical physicians.
- 50-80% of the patients treated in medical clinics have a diagnosable psychiatric illness and 10-20% of medical patients suffer primarily from an emotional disorder.
- 50% of patients in psychiatric clinic populations have undiagnosed medical conditions.
- 10% of self-referred psychiatric patients have symptoms which are due solely to a medical illness.

<u>Always</u> evaluate psychiatric patients medically. Be particularly alert to patients presenting with depression, confusion, memory loss, anxiety, personality changes, psychosis of rapid onset, visual hallucinations, and illusions. Always be suspicious of symptoms of sudden onset in a patient, particularly over 35 years old, who previously has been problem-free. Recognize that patients (or their physicians) often can identify a "precipitating event" for even the most organic of psychiatric conditions - don't be fooled.

<u>Always</u> consider psychiatric possibilities for physical symptoms in medical patients. Take a good history including past emotional problems. Why is the patient coming for help now?

PSYCHIATRIC SYMPTOMS:

There are only a few typical psychiatric presentations and many different medical illnesses which can cause them. Some of the most common associations are listed below although almost any physical condition can contribute to symptom production.

Presentation	Disease
Anxiety	hyperthyroidism hypoglycemia pneumonia acute intermittent porphyria pheochromocytoma mitral valve prolapse angina pectoris cardiac arrhythmias hyper- and hypoparathyroidism hypothyroidism Cushing's Disease menstrual irregularities
Depression	hypothyroidism debilitating disease pneumonia, other infections Cushing's Disease Addison's Disease pancreatic carcinoma intracranial tumors Pernicious Anemia hyper- and hypoparathyroidism
Confusion, memory loss	Numerous medical conditions (see chapters 5 and 6)
Mixed psychotic- hysterical symptoms	MS Wilson's Disease SLE intracranial tumors hyperthyroidism psychomotor epilepsy general paresis Huntington's Chorea metachromatic leukodystrophy porphyria

MEDICAL DISEASES:

No medical illness produces pathognomonic psychiatric symptoms yet each has a typical <u>range</u> of presentations. Some of the most characteristic are listed below but more comprehensive sources are available (eg, Lishman, 1978; Jefferson and Marshall, 1981). In many of these diseases, the patient develops psychiatric pathology before any medical signs or symptoms are noticed.

Endocrine:

Hyperthyroidism - anxiety, restlessness, emotional
lability, wt loss, sweating, fine tremor, atypical
depression with confusion in older patients.

Hypothyroidism - depression, fatigue, apathy, occasionally anxiety and psychosis ("myxedema madness"), dry
skin, EEG slowing, cold intolerance.

Hyperparathyroidism - anxiety and irritability; depression,
apathy, and fatigue; confusion and delirium; abdominal
and bone pain, kidney stones, duodenal ulcer.
Symptoms progress to psychosis and coma as the serum
calcium levels rise.

Hypoparathyroidism - similar to hyper- but with anxiety
and emotional lability more common; seizures, tetany.

Hypoadrenalism (Addison's Disease) - fatigue, apathy,
depression, weakness, occasional confusion.

Pheochromocytoma - anxiety, restlessness, apprehension
and panic, flushing, headaches; all during attacks.

Hypoglycemia - symptoms vary with blood sugar; episodic
anxiety, tremor, sweating, personality changes,
bizarre behavior.

Diabetes Mellitus - depression, apathy, confusion,
intellectual dullness.

Premenstrual Syndrome (PMS) - as many as 25% of women
develop significant physical/psychological discomfort
during the 4-5 days prior to menses, ending shortly
after flow begins. Common symptoms include irritability, tension, tearfulness, moderate depression, a
sense of bloating, swelling of the extremities, and
headaches, but may include more severe symptoms such
as profound depression, aggressiveness, and even
psychosis. The etiology is unknown but may be related
to hormonal imbalance: possibly prolactin, estrogen,
or prostaglandins. Women with a primary affective
disorder may be at risk for problems. No treatment is
certain but progestogenic oral contraceptives,
bromocriptine, Li, and/or psychotherapy may help.

Infections:

Depression, anxiety, OBS, and acute psychoses all can
occur due to a variety of infectious processes, depending
upon the patient's sensitivity, his age and physical
condition, the site of the infection, and the agent.
Particularly common are symptoms with pneumonia
(particularly delirium with bacterial and depression with
viral), infectious mononucleosis (anxiety and psychosis may
be the first symptoms of mono; depression is common late),
viral hepatitis (the posthepatitic syndrome - weakness,
irritability, lethargy, depression), syphilis (general
paresis), and TB.

Other:

Acute Intermittent Porphyria - 15% of cases present first with psychiatric symptoms; anxiety, irritability, emotional outbursts, depression, acute psychosis; abdominal pain, peripheral neuropathies and bulbar palsies, vomiting and constipation.

Hepatolenticular degeneration (Wilson's Disease) - May present with a labile mood, explosive outbursts, and psychotic behavior in a young man before the development of cirrhosis, portal hypertension, rigidity, Kayser-Fleischer rings, and dementia.

Pellagra - dementia, diarrhea, and dermatitis; also depression, personality changes, and a confusional psychosis.

Systemic lupus erythematosis (SLE) - Patient may present with confusion, an affective state, and psychotic behavior before physical signs appear.

Pernicious Anemia - depression and fatigue but also an organic psychosis. Look at blood for characteristic megaloblastic anemia.

Pancreatic carcinoma - severe depression in some patients.

Prolapse of the mitral valve - frequently presents as generalized anxiety disorder, panic disorder, or agoraphobia with panic attacks.

REFERENCES

1. Abramowitz ES, Baker AH, Fleischer SF: Onset of depressive psychiatric crises and the menstrual cycle. Am J Psychiat 139:475, 1982.
2. Cohen SI: Cushings syndrome: a psychiatric study of 29 patients. Brit J Psychiat 136:120, 1980.
3. Cox JL, Connor Y, Kendell RE: Prospective study of the psychiatric disorders of childbirth. Brit J Psychiat 140:111, 1982.
4. Crowe RR, Pauls DL, Slymen DJ, Noyes R: A family study of anxiety neurosis. Arch Gen Psychiat 37:77, 1980.
5. Hall RCW: Psychiatric Presentations of Medical Illness. New York, SP Med & Scientific Books, 1983.
6. Hall RCW: Psychiatric effects of thyroid hormone disturbance. Psychosomatics 24:7, 1983.
7. Hall RCW, Popkin MK, Devaul RA, Faillace LA, Stickney SK: Physical illness presenting as psychiatric disease. Arch Gen Psychiat 35:1315, 1978.
8. Jefferson JW, Marshall JR: Neuropsychiatric Features of Medical Disorders. New York, Plenum Med Book Co, 1981.

9. Kantor JS, Zitrin CM, Zeldis SM: Mitral valve prolapse
    syndrome in agoraphobic patients. Am J Psychiat
    137:467, 1980.
10. Kelly WF, Checkley SA, Bender DA, Mashiter K: Cushing's
    syndrome and depression - a prospective study of 26
    patients. Brit J Psychiat 140:1194, 1983.
11. Korami EK: Physical Illness in the Psychiatric Patient.
    Springfield, Ill, CC Thomas, 1982.
12. Levenson AJ, Hall RCW: Neuropsychiatric Manifestations
    of Physical Disease in the Elderly. New York, Raven Pr,
    1981.
13. Lishman WA: Organic Psychiatry. Oxford, Blackwell Pub,
    1978.
14. Massey EW: Neuropsychiatric manifestations of porphyria.
    J Clin Psychiat 41:208, 1980.
15. Reich P, Regestein QR, Murawski BJ, DeSilva RA, Lown B:
    Unrecognized organic mental disorders in survivors of
    cardiac arrest. Am J Psychiat 140:1194, 1983.
16. Rubinow DR, Roy-Byren P: Premenstrual syndromes:
    overview from a methodologic perspective. Am J Psychiat
    141:163, 1984.
17. Silberfarb PM, Greer S: Psychological concomitants of
    cancer. Am J Psychotherapy 36:470, 1982.

Chapter 15

Psychiatric Presentations of Neurological Disease

Many of the psychiatric symptoms caused by various neurological diseases (eg, CNS tumor, trauma, seizure, infection) can be correlated directly to the CNS site involved.

Frontal lobes:

Prefrontal damage – the frontal lobe syndrome occurs with unilateral or bilateral damage (personality changes, irritability, euphoria, apathy, pseudodepression, impulsivity, social inappropriateness). Do not mistake for depression or mania. Intelligence is usually unimpaired in unilateral damage. Symptoms are milder if only one side is involved.

If the premotor area is involved (on left), there may also be apraxia of the left hand and Broca's (expressive) aphasia. Don't confuse with psychosis.

Temporal lobes:

Stimulation or lesions may produce visual and olfactory hallucinations, non-complex auditory hallucinations, and aggressive psychotic behavior.
Dominant lobe lesion may produce Wernicke's aphasia.
Nondominant lobe lesion may produce agnosia for sounds, intonations, and music.
Bilateral lesions may produce the amnestic disorder of Korsakoff and the Kluver-Bucy Syndrome (placidity and hypersexuality).

Parietal lobes:

Dominant lobe lesions may produce language difficulties (eg, inability to express or understand spoken words, perform simple tasks, read, and/or write), tactile agnosia, apraxia, and intellectual deterioration.
Nondominant lobe lesions may produce anosognosia.

120

Occipital lobes:

Some lesions produce crude, flashing visual illusions and hallucinations.

Limbic system:

Effects are diverse but usually involve primitive and emotional behavior - eg, emotional lability, fear, rage, impulsivity, depression, memory loss. Also amnestic syndrome when mamillary bodies involved (Korsakoff's Syndrome).

NEUROLOGICAL DISEASES:

Neurological disorders can produce a variety of psychiatric symptoms - consult a comprehensive source for detailed descriptions of specific conditions (eg, Lishman, 1978). Some major diseases are presented below.

Parkinson's Disease - frequently accompanied by apathy and depression.

Huntington's Chorea - may present first with psychiatric symptoms (eg, emotional lability, impulsiveness, depression, hallucinations, delusions). Don't mistake for schizophrenia, major depression, or mania. Look for family history, movement disorder, and dementia.

Multiple sclerosis (MS) - early psychiatric symptoms are common, particularly emotional lability, euphoria, transient psychotic episodes, depression, and an "hysterical" presentation.

Intracranial tumors - 50% of patients develop psychiatric symptoms and occasionally they may be the presenting symptoms. Pattern is site-related although there is usually a degree of generalized OBS. Early personality changes are often subtle - "He's not the same person anymore." Aphasias due to tumor (or any other cause) may mimic psychotic language disorders - there are qualitative differences between these two types of speech.

Head trauma - a post-concussion syndrome includes irritability, emotional lability, and personality changes.

CNS infection - typically presents with OBS (usually irritability and restlessness initially). General paresis (CNS syphilis) usually presents as a gradually

developing dementia but can produce a variety of
confusing symptoms - eg, may mimic schizophrenia,
mania, depression, somatization disorder.

GILLES DE LA TOURETTE SYNDROME (DSM-III p 76, 307.23) -
This neuropsychiatric syndrome of uncertain etiology
usually develops in latency or early adolescence with
the onset of one or more poorly controlled symptoms
including head or extremity tics, eyeblinks, and the
spasmodic production of coughs or grunts which
occasionally can include verbal obscenities
(coprolalia). This disorder is often severe and
lifelong, occurs (along with other tic phenomena) with
increased incidence in families, and has an apparent
genetic component. All symptoms are worsened by
stress and may be improved by psychotherapy, but
primary treatment is pharmacological: haloperidol (the
mainstay; 80-90% of patients improve; 2-12 mg/day),
clonidine (0.1-0.5 mg/day; see Cohen et al, 1980),
pimozide (2-12 mg/day; see Shapiro et al, 1983).
Stimulant medication can precipitate or worsen
Tourette symptoms and must be avoided.

REFERENCES

1. Benson DF, Blumer D: Psychiatric Aspects of
    Neurological Disease. New York, Grune & Stratton, 1975.
2. Caine ED, Shoulson I: Psychiatric syndromes in
    Huntington's disease. Am J Psychiat 140:728, 1983.
3. Cohen DJ: Detlor J, Young JG, Shaywitz BA: Clonidine
    ameliorates Gilles de la Tourette Syndrome. Arch Gen
    Psychiat 37:1350, 1980.
4. Flor-Henry P: Cerebral Basis of Psychopathology.
    Boston, John Wright, 1983.
5. Hamilton NG, Frick RB, Takahashi T, Hopping MW:
    Psychiatric symptoms and cerebellar pathology. Am J
    Psychiat 140:1322, 1983.
6. Heath RG, Franklin DE, Shraberg D: Gross pathology of
    the cerebellum in patients diagnosed and treated as
    functional psychiatric disorders. J Nerv Ment Dis
    167:585, 1979.
7. Heilman KM, Valenstein E: Emotional disorders caused by
    CNS dysfunction. Geriatrics 35:77, January, 1980.
8. Kertesz A: Aphasia and Associated Disorders. New York,
    Grune & Stratton, 1979.
9. Lishman WA: Organic Psychiatry. Oxford, Blackwell Pub,
    1978.
10. Lowe TL, Cohen DJ, Detlor J, Kremenitzer MW, Shaywitz
    BA: Stimulant medications precipitate Tourette's
    syndrome. JAMA 247:1729, 1982.

11. Nasrallah HA, McChesney CM: Psychopathology of corpus callosum tumors. Biol Psychiat 16:663, 1981.
12. Pauls DL, Cohen DJ, Heimbuch R, Detlor J, Kidd KK: Familial pattern and transmission of Gilles de la Tourette syndrome and multiple tics. Arch Gen Psychiat 38:1091, 1981.
13. Pincus JH, Tucker GJ: Behavioral Neurology. New York, Oxford Univ Pr, 1978.
14. Rickler KC: Neurological diagnosis in psychiatric disease. Psychiatic Ann 13:408, 1983.
15. Schiffer RB: Psychiatric aspects of clinical neurology. Am J Psychiat 140:205, 1983.
16. Shapiro AK, Shapiro E, Eisenkraft GJ: Treatment of Gilles de la Tourette syndrome with pimozide. Am J Psychiat 140:1183, 1983.
17. Shapiro AK, Shapiro E: An update on Tourette syndrome. Am J Psychotherapy 36:379, 1982.

Chapter 16

Psychiatry of Alcohol

Alcohol is the major substance of abuse. 68% of Americans drink, 12% are heavy drinkers (men 2:1), 10 million have alcohol abuse problems, and 50% of homicides and auto deaths are alcohol-related. Certain populations are at risk: eg, urban blacks, some Indian tribes, bartenders.

CLASSIFICATION

Normal (recreational) drinking grades into pathological use. ALCOHOL ABUSE (DSM-III p 169, 305.0) is diagnosed if there is at least one month of impaired social and occupational functioning due to alcohol use. Individual patterns can vary from continuous consumption to periodic binges but all demonstrate the inability to abstain from drinking or to stop drinking once started. Such drinking usually results in depression and anxiety. Beginning often as evening and weekend drinking, the pattern usually becomes established by the late 20's in males (later in females) with gradual deterioration in some during their 30's and 40's. Spontaneous remissions can occur. Blackouts (anterograde amnesia for events that occurred during acute intoxication but while conscious and quite functional) often follow more severe drinking.

If the patient also demonstrates tolerance (increased amounts needed to achieve effect) or withdrawal, he has ALCOHOL DEPENDENCE (ALCOHOLISM) (DSM-III p 169, 303.9). Broader definitions of alcoholism are used by some; eg, "patients with significant impairment due to persistent and excessive alcohol use, possibly involving physiological, psychological, or social dysfunction" (AMA Manual of Alcoholism). The etiology of alcoholism is unknown.

Adoption studies indicate a genetic factor in some families - increased frequency of alcohol abuse and

124

sociopathy among male and possible increase of depression among female relatives of alcoholics. Cultural groups are differentially affected (eg, low among Jews and Orientals). All social strata are affected - fewer than 5% are "skid row" types. There is no "typical alcoholic personality" yet many alcoholics are immature and overdependent, have a low tolerance for frustration, and experience chronic anxiety. Patients with chronic anxiety, mood disorders (particularly females), schizophrenia, dementia, and antisocial personality disorder are at risk to "self-medicate" with alcohol. Always rule out these primary psychiatric disorders.

RECOGNIZING THE ALCOHOLIC

The majority of alcohol abusers go unrecognized by physicians until their social and occupational life and their physical health have been significantly harmed. Early recognition is important. These patients frequently conceal alcohol use - keep a high index of suspicion. Be suspicious if the predominant complaints include:

1. chronic anxiety and tension
2. insomnia
3. chronic depression
4. headaches, blackouts
5. nausea and vomiting, vague GI problems
6. tachycardia, palpitations
7. frequent falls or minor injuries

Ask about absenteeism, job loss, financial difficulties, family trouble. Ask, "Do you drink?" Be encouraging and non-judgemental. Get drinking specifics (number of beers/day, oz/glass, drink alone?, etc). Interview relatives and friends, if possible.

Chronic drinking frequently elevates serum gamma-glutamyltransferase (GGT) and RBC MCV. These measures, coupled with evidence of more acute alcoholic insult (protein, Alk Phos, LDH, SGOT, SGPT, etc - see Eckardt et al, 1981) constitute a fairly reliable laboratory screen for alcoholism.

CLINICAL PRESENTATIONS

When presenting acutely, always determine the patient's recent drinking history:

1. Is he currently intoxicated?
2. Time since last drink?

Intoxication Syndromes

ALCOHOL INTOXICATION (DSM-III p 129, 303.00): Alcohol is a CNS depressant which initially disinhibits, then depresses. Early intoxication includes liveliness, a sense of well-being, and a smell of alcohol on the breath (blood alcohol levels up to 100 mg/100 ml); grading into irritability, emotional lability, and incoordination (100-150 mg%); which grades into apathy, slurred speech, and ataxia (150-250 mg%); which can become alcoholic coma (above 250-400 mg%; an emergency - get blood alcohol level and check for presence of other drugs; treat with intubation, CPR, etc, if necessary). Blood alcohol levels vary with drinking experience and thus are only approximate.

Acute intoxication can mimic schizophrenia, mania, depression, hysteria, etc, so delay detailed interview and final diagnosis until patient is sober. Evaluate carefully for medical problems (see below) - differential includes hypoglycemia, CNS infection, and toxic psychosis of other etiology. Intoxicated patients may be uncooperative, assaultive, and dangerous - be civil, nonthreatening, accepting, respectful, patient, but prepared with force. Attempt non-pharmacological management (quiet room, support, coffee) but sedation may be necessary: eg, diazepam 5-20 mg PO or IM (erratically absorbed), but be cautious of over-sedation. Decide if the patient just needs to "sleep it off," is at risk for withdrawal, or is becoming comatose. Should he go home with family, be observed overnight, be hospitalized, or go to jail? Be familiar with community resources.

ALCOHOL IDIOSYNCRATIC INTOXICATION (Pathological Intoxication) (DSM-III p 132, 291.40) is an unusual and controversial condition of marked aggressiveness and emotional lability, occasionally of psychotic proportions, which follows ingestion of small quantities of alcohol in an otherwise normal person. Etiology is unknown. Some patients retain this pattern for life. Episodes appear suddenly and may last for hours or a day or more, often with amnesia for the episode afterward. Sedate (benzodiazepines, Haldol) and control until sober. Rule out temporal lobe epilepsy. Alcoholic paranoia has a similar presentation but with strong paranoid delusions. It usually occurs in chronic alcoholics who are actively drinking.

Alcohol Withdrawal Syndromes

These may occur in heavy drinkers or alcoholics who stop drinking or who just reduce their consumption. Don't overlook them in the "closet" alcoholic - eg, the business-

man or housewife who temporarily abstains while in the
hospital for other reasons. If the patient is withdrawing,
delay final diagnostic conclusions.

ALCOHOL WITHDRAWAL (DSM-III p 133, 291.80) - tremulousness,
weakness, nausea and vomiting, "dry heaves," anxiety,
insomnia and bad dreams, mild illusions and hallucinations,
hypervigilance, paresthesias, numbness, tinnitus, and/or
blurred vision beginning within the first 12-18 hours of
reduced drinking. Symptoms disappear with further
drinking, leading to a vicious cycle. Debilitated,
medically ill patients are at risk. Alcoholic convulsions
(generalized, self-limited, single or in small groups)
occur in some, usually in the first two days of withdrawal,
but sometimes later. If the seizure is focal - suspect CNS
pathology (eg, subdural).

ALCOHOL WITHDRAWAL DELIRIUM (Delirium Tremens - DTs) (DSM-
III p 134, 291.00) is a life-threatening delirium with
disorientation, agitation, memory disturbances, hallucinations (usually visual, but also tactile, auditory, vestibu-
lar, etc), delusions, powerful autonomic discharge (hypertension, tachycardia, sweating), tremor, ataxia, and fever
beginning 2-8 days after reduced drinking. Tremulousness
and seizures can precede, and often are mistaken for, the
much less common DTs. Malnourishment and medical illness
increases the risk of delirium. Mortality rate is 10-15%
for the complete syndrome (often from secondary infection
or acute heart failure).

ALCOHOLIC HALLUCINOSIS (DSM-III p 135, 291.30) displays
striking auditory hallucinations (voices, sounds) and mixed
other withdrawal symptoms (mild tremor, anger,
apprehension) but the patient typically has a clear
sensorium and is oriented. It usually occurs in the first
three days after cessation of drinking in patients who have
had years of heavy drinking. Patients may be dangerous or
self-destructive while hallucinating. Usually self-limited
(within one week), occasional cases last for months or
become chronic (chronic alcoholic hallucinosis).
Differential includes alcoholic paranoia and toxic
psychosis (amphetamine, cocaine). Differentiation from
paranoid schizophrenia is difficult in chronic cases (look
for other signs of schizophrenia).

COMPLICATIONS OF CHRONIC ALCOHOLISM

        Chronic alcoholics have numerous complicating
diseases.

<u>Medical:</u> gastritis, gastric ulcer, diarrhea, anemia,
hypertension, pancreatitis, cirrhosis (in less than
10% of alcoholics - alcohol plus poor diet),
persistent impotence, insomnia.

<u>Neurological:</u>
  1. Peripheral neuropathy (vitamin B deficiencies)
  2. Alcoholic cerebellar degeneration
  3. Central pontine myelinolysis
  4. Marchiafava-Bignami Disease
  5. Cerebral atrophy
  6. Alcoholic myopathy and cardiomyopathy
  7. Wernicke's Encephalopathy (vertical and horizontal
     nystagmus, sixth nerve palsies, ataxia, and
     confusion) - due to thiamine deficiency (give 50 mg
     IV and 50 mg IM, then 50 mg IM daily until patient
     is eating). An emergency - if treated early, it
     usually quickly clears.

<u>Psychiatric:</u>
  1. <u>ALCOHOL AMNESTIC DISORDER</u> (<u>Korsakoff's Disease</u>)
     (DSM-III p 136, 291.10) is a profound recent short-
     term memory loss (retrograde and anterograde) with
     confabulation, which follows untreated Wernicke's
     Encephalopathy or develops insidiously. Typically,
     events are remembered for several minutes (ie,
     immediate memory is OK) and then are forgotten. Due
     to thiamine deficiency - lesions in the mammillary
     bodies and thalamus. Treat as in Wernicke's Disease.
     Impairment is often life-long, yet 75% improve with
     time.
  2. <u>DEMENTIA ASSOCIATED WITH ALCOHOLISM</u> (DSM-III p 137,
     291.2) refers to a dementia (ie, all intellectual
     functions affected), ranging from mild to severe,
     following many years of alcohol abuse and with no
     other obvious etiology. Few alcoholics are affected
     and the predisposition is unknown.
  3. Suicide
  4. Drug Abuse

<u>Other:</u>
  1. Fetal Alcohol Syndrome describes small, hyperactive,
     retarded children with variable anatomical
     abnormalities including ptosis, epicanthal folds,
     hypoplastic maxilla, cleft lip and palate,
     microcephaly, and hypospadias. Although not
     definite, it is thought to be due to a teratogenic
     effect on the fetus by alcohol consumed by the
     mother while pregnant. It is one of the most common
     causes of retardation.

TREATMENT OF WITHDRAWAL

Treatment varies with the severity of the symptoms.
When in doubt, hospitalize temporarily, however, many
patients manifesting mild withdrawal symptoms can be
treated in a supportive environment, with good nutrition,
and without medication.

1. Be clear and unambiguous. Identify yourself. Explain
   procedures. Place patient in a lighted room. Include
   family and familiar people. Use restraints if needed.
   Keep under constant observation.

2. Carefully evaluate (PE, chest X-ray, chemistry,
   electrolytes including calcium and magnesium, CBC, PT,
   occult blood in stool, occasionally an LP). Incidence
   of complicating disorders is high - eg, pneumonia, TB,
   UTIs, hypoglycemia, diabetic ketoacidosis, anemia,
   shock, gastritis with hematemesis, acute hemorrhagic
   pancreatitis, cirrhosis and hepatic failure, meningitis. Be particularly careful to exclude (1) a
   subdural hematoma due to a fall and (2) withdrawal
   from other substances. Treat these conditions if
   present.

3. Use medication - to assure sleep, prevent exhaustion,
   reduce agitation. Sedate until calm (but avoid
   oversedation) then taper over 4-8 days (ie, decrease
   by approximately 20% of total first day's dose each
   day). The delirium often resolves within one day.
   Benzodiazepines currently are preferred but chloral
   hydrate, paraldehyde, and barbiturates are also
   useful. Phenothiazines lower seizure threshold, but
   may be useful with chronic psychotics and alcoholic
   hallucinosis.

   Tremulousness: eg, chlordiazepoxide 25-50 mg PO,
      q4-6 hr until comfortable.
   Delirium: eg, chlordiazepoxide 50-100 mg, PO or IM
      every hr until calm (able to stay in bed), then
      q4 hrs. IM doses are often poorly absorbed - can
      lead to early undersedation, then cumulative
      oversedation. If patient is severe, give IV
      slowly.

4. If withdrawal seizures persist, consider 5-10 mg of
   diazepam slowly by IV or 100-150 mg of phenobarbital
   IM. If a primary seizure disorder exists, begin
   diphenylhydantoin.

5. Give Thiamine 100 mg IM, then 50 mg PO TID X 4 days. Also provide a high carbohydrate diet and multi-vitamins daily.

6. Correct fluid and electrolyte imbalances - particularly hypokalemia (replace carefully over 24 hr or longer via IV) and hypomagnesemia (may exacerbate seizures - give magnesium sulfate 2-4 ml of 50% solution IM q6 hr X 2 days).

7. Record pulse, BP, and temp every half-hour initially. Treat shock with fluids, whole blood, and vasopressors.

8. Check for and treat: Hypoglycemia, prolonged PT (give Vitamin K 10 mg IM), fever (aspirin, sponge baths - rule out superimposed infection).

9. Anxiety, irritability, depression, and insomnia may persist for weeks after the acute episode - a vulnerable period for the alcoholic. Anti-anxiety agents may be of use for 1-2 weeks.

TREATMENT OF ALCOHOLISM

Successful treatment of alcoholism is difficult but not hopeless. However, there is no definitive treatment.

1. Identify its presence. Get your facts straight (family drinking history, recent intake).
2. Develop a personal rapport with the patient - be warm and supportive but firm. Be open and matter-of-fact about the drinking but insist on abstinence. Encourage patient to maintain employment and social involvement.
3. Treat all medical complications of drinking.
4. Treat any complicating primary psychiatric illness (eg, schizophrenia, affective disorder, anxiety disorder). If the patient is likely to drink, recognize that tricyclics potentiate the CNS depressant effect of alcohol and that alcohol can promote lithium toxicity.
5. Enlist family members in treatment. Evaluate family's contribution to the problem. Consider family therapy; marital therapy.
5. Consider disulfiram (Antabuse) use in cooperative but backsliding patients. It inhibits aldehyde dehydrogenase leading to toxic acetaldehyde build-up 15-30 minutes after alcohol consumption, which leads to anxiety and apprehension, sweating, nausea and vomiting, tachycardia, headache, and hypotension. Give 500 mg PO QD X 1 wk, then maintain on 250 mg daily (range 125-500 mg). Carefully inform patient of the possible reactions. Effects last up to two weeks

after last dose, however not every patient shows an Antabuse reaction. Occasional adverse effects include sedation, a metallic taste, mild GI disturbances, mild ataxia, and a peripheral neuropathy. Question its use in thoroughly irresponsible patients - hepatotoxicity and toxic psychoses can occur and severe reactions (to a large alcohol challenge) can lead to shock and coma. Contraindicated in patients with unstable medical conditions or histories of psychosis, OBS, MI, or heart failure. Biggest problem with disulfiram - patients stop taking it so they can drink.

7. Group therapy appears to be the most effective technique. In most cases, work with or refer patient to a specialized multidisciplinary treatment team. Make referral personally, with the patient present. AA (Alcoholics Anonymous) can help - encourage patient's consideration. Also useful: Alanon (spouses of alcoholics). Hospitalize in an alcohol unit (milieu therapy) if even temporary sobriety cannot be achieved.

8. Be patient. Keep trying.

REFERENCES

1. Butters N, Cermak LS: Alcoholic Korsakoff's Syndrome. New York, Academic Pr, 1980.
2. Cadoret RJ, Colleen AC, Grove WM: Development of alcoholism in adoptees raised apart from alcoholic biologic relatives. Arch Gen Psychiat 37:561, 1980.
3. Eckardt MJ, Ryback RS, Rawlings RR, Graubard BI: Biochemical diagnosis of alcoholism. JAMA 246:2707, 1981.
4. Goodwin DW: Alcoholism and heredity. Arch Gen Psychiat 36:57, 1979.
5. Hayes SL: Ethanol and oral diazepam absorption. NEJM 296:186, 1977.
6. Hollender MH: Pathological intoxication - Is there such an entity?. J Clin Psychiat 32:426, 1979.
7. Greenblatt DJ, Shader RI: Treatment of the alcohol withdrawal syndrome, in Shader RI: Manual of Psychiatric Therapeutics. Boston, Little Brown & Co, 1975.
8. Lewis CE, Rice J, Helzer JE: Diagnostic interactions: alcoholism and antisocial personality. J Nerv Ment Dis 171:105, 1983.
9. Loosen PT, Wilson IC, Dew BW, Tipermas A: Thyrotropin-releasing hormone (TRH) in abstinent alcoholic men. Am J Psychiat 140:1145, 1983.

10. Papoz L, Warnet JM, Pequignot G et at: Alcohol consumption in a healthy population: relationship to gamma-glutamyltransferase activity and mean corpuscular volume. JAMA 245: 1748, 1981.
11. Pollock VE, Volavka J, Goodwin DW, Mednick SA, Gabrielli Wf, Knop J, Schulsinger F: The EEG after alcohol administration in men at risk for alcoholism. Arch Gen Psychiat 40:857, 1983.
12. Vaillant GE, Milofsky ES: Natural history of male alcoholism. Arch Gen Psychiat 39:127, 1982.
13. Whitfield CL et al: Detoxification of 1,024 alcoholic patients without psychoactive drugs. JAMA 239:1409, 1978.
14. Yudofsky SC, Stevens L, Silver J, Barsa J, Williams D: Propranolol in the treatment of rage and violent behavior associated with Korsakoff's psychosis. Am J Psychiat 141:114, 1984.

Chapter 17

Psychiatry of Drug Abuse

Drug abusers are common, often unrecognized, and poorly understood. There is great variability in the degree of drug use from patient to patient. Abuse occurs if the patient has (1) been using drugs for more than one month, (2) has difficulty controlling his use, and (3) has impaired social and/or occupational functioning because of that use. Drug dependence requires the presence of either tolerance or withdrawal. Patients may be classified by the type of drug abused (see below) or by the pattern and reason for abuse. Some recognized patterns of use (abuse) include:

- Recreational use - Patient takes drugs for "fun" and is not physically or psychologically dependent upon them. He may also take them "just to be part of the group" or because it is a counter-cultural requirement.
- Iatrogenic addiction - Patient addicted "by mistake." Patient (and physician) may or may not recognize the addiction. Many of these patients are convinced that they must have the drug to function (eg, to sleep, to interact with others) and may go to great lengths to talk their physicians into prescribing medication.
- The chronic drug addict - These patients usually abuse "street" drugs. Many have underlying depressions. Many have antisocial personalities. Some take drugs in an effort to self-medicate a chronic psychiatric disorder (eg, major depression, schizophrenia).

Abusers are not "all alike" but they do have many common features including the frequent presence of marked depression and anxiety, increased dependency needs (often hidden), low self-esteem, and a chronic course resistant to treatment. Also, evaluate for psychiatric illness.

Treatment of chronic drug abusers is difficult - frequently an inpatient setting is required. Whether inpatients or outpatients, drug abusers should be treated

firmly but with support and understanding. Set clear
limits and stick to them. Insist on dealing with the
patient only when he is not intoxicated. Be reasonably
confrontive. You will be tested and manipulated by many
patients - don't respond with retribution. Follow many of
the pri..ciples used in dealing with the alcoholic patient
(see chapter 16).

The most common drugs of abuse, their clinical
presentations, and treatment follow. Multiple drug abusers
are common.

OPIOIDS

DRUGS INVOLVED:

opium
morphine
diacetylmorphine (Heroin, horse, smack)
methadone
codeine
oxycodone (eg, Percodan, in mixture)
hydromorphone (Dilaudid)
levorphanol (Levo-Dromoran)
pentazocine (Talwin)
meperidine (Demerol)
propoxyphene (Darvon)

Some of these compounds are naturally occurring (opium
and its constituents morphine and codeine) while the others
are semi-synthetic or wholly synthetic. Some of these
drugs have legitimate uses (eg, morphine, meperidine) while
others are solely substances of abuse (eg, heroin). Most
are obtained illegally "on the street" and are used
primarily by a young, lower socioeconomic population while
others are abused more widely (eg, Demerol, Dilaudid, and
Percodan are common drugs of abuse among professionals).
Common routes of administration are IV (heroin, morphine,
methadone - "mainlining"), SC (Heroin, meperidine -"skin
popping"), nasally (heroin - "snorting"), orally
(methadone, Percodan), and smoked (opium). It is
frequently very difficult to determine the daily dose used
because (1) the abuser often over-estimates the dose and
(2) the amount of active drug in a "bag" bought on the
street is uncertain. Frequently a bag of heroin is 95%
adulterants (eg, quinine, mannitol, lactose).

Abuse (OPIOID ABUSE, DSM-III p 172, 305.5) and
dependency (OPIOID DEPENDENCE, DSM-III p 172, 304.0) are
common in some populations and the search for drugs or

money for drugs accounts for the majority of the crime in
some communities. Some people (less than 50%) are able to
abuse opioids without becoming dependent (ie, without
tolerance and/or withdrawal) and they often are used
recreationally without addiction. Those persons who become
dependent represent a high risk group.

- 1% of all heroin addicts in the USA die each year. Most
  common cause is an inadvertently fatal OD - eg, an
  addict using "bags" of 5% heroin accidently buys a
  supply containing 15% heroin. Also common is death
  during violent crime.
- The majority of addicts have a personality disorder -
  usually antisocial type. They also have a high
  incidence of depression and anxiety. Suicide rate is
  elevated.
- Heroin addicts are at markedly increased risk (due to
  dirty needles, poor nutrition, etc) for developing
  certain medical illnesses.

  hepatitis, serum and infectious
  subacute bacterial endocarditis
  tetanus
  pneumonia; pulmonary edema, embolus, abscess; TB
  cellulitis, thrombophlebitis, septicemia
  UTIs, glomerulonephritis, nephrosis
  osteomyelitis
  transverse myelitis
  polyneuropathy (Guillain-Barre type)
  VD
  nasal septum perforation (due to "snorting")
  needle "tracts" on the arms (and legs)

  Always carefully evaluate hospitalized addicts
medically. Recognize that the analgesic properties of the
opioids may obscure acute medical problems. The majority
of addicts "grow out of" their habit over the years (or
die), thus there are relatively few older abusers.

  Treatment of the opioid addict usually means treatment
of the acute episodes (eg, intoxication and withdrawal -
see below). "Cure" of the addiction does occur in some
well motivated patients yet most addicts continue their
abuse over at least several years. The two major forms of
long-term treatment (both with equivocal results) are:

1. Methadone Maintenance - Patients are maintained as outpatients on daily doses of methadone of 40-120 mg.
   This level controls the craving for (and eliminates
   the euphoria from) heroin. The patient can then
   develop some skills, hold a job, go to school, etc. -

and can often profit from intensive psychotherapy.
Poorly motivated patients may succeed by this route.
LAAM, a chemical congener of methadone, has recently
found use as a long-acting replacement for methadone
(patient takes it 3X/wk).

2. Residential, drug-free, self-help programs - Patients
   (usually highly motivated) stay 1-2 years (or more) in
   a close "therapeutic community" which insists on the
   drug-free state and on personal responsibility.
   Confrontation and behavior modification are frequently
   used. Poor "candidates" usually drop out.

The two major features of illicit opioid use which
bring patients to medical attention are intoxication (and
overdosage) and withdrawal.

OPIOID INTOXICATION (DSM-III p 142, 305.50) develops
rapidly after an IV dose (1-5 minutes). The time course
varies with the drug used.

Drug	Duration of action (hrs)
heroin	4 - 6
methadone	12 - 24
meperidine	2 - 4

The abstinence syndrome begins after this period of time in
the dependent patient. It is because of these kinetics
that many heroin addicts "shoot up" 3-4 X/day, or more.

Symptoms are similar for most of the narcotics.

Psychological symptoms - a "rush" immediately follows IV
administration (described as a "whole body orgasm"
with the focus in the abdomen). This is accompanied
by euphoria and a sense of well-being or dysphoria
(usually anxiety and fear), a drowsiness and "nodding
off," apathy, psychomotor retardation, and difficulty
concentrating.

Physical symptoms - miosis (pupillary constriction),
slurred speech, respiratory depression, hypotension,
hypothermia, bradycardia, constipation, and nausea and
vomiting. Skin ulcers are common with meperidine
injection. Seizures may occur in the patient tolerant
to meperidine.

An overdose (either accidental or intentional) is a
medical emergency - these patients may die of respiratory
depression and pulmonary edema. Look for needle tracts and
pinpoint pupils in the unconscious patient but recognize
that if the patient already has experienced significant CNS

anoxia, the pupils may be dilated. Seizures occasionally occur (particularly with meperidine).

Treat the OD with intensive medical care (ICU) and the narcotic antagonist, naloxone (Narcan). Give 0.4 mg IV and repeat X 5 at 3 minute intervals. Expect a rapid response (ie, clearing in 1-2 minutes) and if this doesn't occur after four doses, suspect another etiology for the coma. If the patient improves, continue monitoring - patient may need additional doses of naloxone since it has a much shorter half-life than either heroin or methadone. Excessive naloxone may throw a dependent patient directly from coma into withdrawal - don't be confused. Multiple drugs may have been taken - be alert to the possibility of a more slowly developing coma from a second agent.

OPIOID WITHDRAWAL (DSM-III p 144, 392.00): In spite of its reputation as a dramatic and traumatic withdrawal syndrome, opioid withdrawal is uncomfortable but usually not life-threatening in healthy young adults and is not nearly as dangerous or difficult to manage as the withdrawal from sedative-hypnotic drugs.

Symptoms are similar for each of the narcotics but the time course varies (dependent partly on the "size of the habit").

Drug	Time after last dose that symptoms begin	Sx peak	Sx disappear
heroin	4 - 8 hrs	1 - 3 days	7 - 10 days
methadone	12 - 48 hrs	4 - 6 days	10 - 21 days
meperidine	2 - 4 hrs	8 - 12 hrs	4 - 5 days

Psychological symptoms - Early there is often intense drug craving followed by severe anxiety, restlessness, irritability, insomnia, and decreased appetite. In this state, the hospitalized patient is frequently extremely demanding and manipulative.

Physical symptoms - Yawning, diaphoresis, tearing, rhinorrhea, pupillary dilation, piloerection (hard to "fake" so look for it), muscle twitching, and hot flashes. Later there is nausea and vomiting, fever, hypertension, tachycardia, tachypnea, diarrhea, and abdominal cramps. Seizures occur with meperidine withdrawal.

Babies born to addicted mothers, including those on methadone maintenance, often experience an abstinence syndrome including a high-pitched cry, irritability, tremor, fever, decreased food intake, vomiting, yawning, and hyperbilirubinemia.

Withdraw these patients gradually by using oral methadone to lessen the symptom severity. After a complete
history and physical (including urine screen for opioids
and other drugs), wait for signs of withdrawal and then
give methadone 10 mg PO. Establish the stabilization dose
over the first 1-2 days by adding 5-10 mg of methadone on a
QID schedule as the patient continues to show signs of
abstinence (recognize that some patients will vigorously
demand more drugs even while they are sedated by their
current dose). Once stabilized, give the methadone on a QD
or BID schedule and reduce the total daily amount by 5
mg/day (or 10-20% of the stabilization dose). Most
withdrawals from heroin addiction take 7-10 days -
methadone addiction withdrawals should be done more slowly
(eg, 2-3 weeks). Alternate methods of opiate withdrawal
using clonidine (Catapres - Gold et al, 1980) or LAAM
(Judson et al, 1983) have recently been developed which
show evidence of being safer and more effective than
methadone withdrawal. Withdraw patients from Talwin using
decreasing doses of Talwin.

If a patient is withdrawing from both opioids and
sedative-hypnotics (not uncommon), concentrate on a safe
sedative-hypnotic withdrawal by maintaining the patient on
10-30 mg of methadone until the first withdrawal has been
completed.

SEDATIVE-HYPNOTICS

DRUGS INVOLVED:

Drug	Dependency-producing Dose (mg/day)
meprobamate (Equanil, Miltown)	1600
methaqualone (Quaalude, Sopor)	600
glutethimide (Doriden)	250
ethchlorvynol (Placidyl)	1000
chloral hydrate (Noctec)	2000
secobarbital (Seconal)	600
pentobarbital (Nembutal)	600
amobarbital (Amytal)	600
chlordiazepoxide (Librium)	300
diazepam (Valium)	60
oxazepam (Serax)	
flurazepam (Dalmane)	
methyprylon (Noludar)	
phenobarbital (Luminal)	

The minimum dependency-producing dose listed above should be considered only approximate - there are individual differences as well as a required period of continuous administration (usually at least 1-3 months) before withdrawal symptoms occur. Oral use is the rule. Street synonyms for some of the sedative-hypnotics include downers, reds, blues, blue velvet, yellows, yellow jackets, sopers, ludes.

CLINICAL SYNDROMES:

The same variety of syndromes occurs with sedative-hypnotic use as occurs with alcohol (see chapter 16). There is cross-tolerance between alcohol and the sedative-hypnotics as well as among the various drugs themselves. The clinical picture varies little from drug to drug although withdrawal phenomena are more severe with the shorter acting drugs and more prolonged with those that have a longer half-life.

SEDATIVE OR HYPNOTIC INTOXICATION (DSM-III p 139, 305.40): Symptoms of intoxication are dose related. Mild intoxica- tion includes a sense of well-being, talkativeness, irrita- bility, and emotional disinhibition. Increased doses produce apathy, confusion, stupor, and coma. Physical signs of intoxication include slurred speech, ataxic gait, incoordination, reduced DTRs, lateral nystagmus, and constricted pupils. Look for fast activity on the EEG. Fatalities are frequent with sedative-hypnotic ODs, usually due to respiratory depression (uncommon with the benzo- diazepines).
Always evaluate sedative-hypnotic abusing patients who present with intoxication for an overt or covert OD. If they are becoming increasingly lethargic, treat as a medical emergency with hospitalization and intensive medical care. Obtain blood and/or urine levels.

SEDATIVE OR HYPNOTIC ABUSE (DSM-III p 170, 305.4): This condition results from the pathological use of one or more of this class of drugs for more than one month. These patients frequently can't abstain from use, once started - a psychological addiction. Abuse of sedative-hypnotics is common and, unlike other substances of abuse, there are two distinct populations and patterns of abuse.

1. Males and females in their teens or 20's who obtain these drugs illegally and use them (as well as many other kinds) for "fun" and to get "high" or to block things out and "get away from the hassle."
2. Middle-aged females who are frequently chronically anxious or depressed and who obtain legal prescrip-

tions from (one or more) physicians for complaints of anxiety and insomnia, gradually increase the dosage themselves in an effort to cope, and often become physiologically addicted. Although these patients are common, they are disproportionately frequently seen by physicians because they ultimately have to "doctor shop" to obtain drugs. Recognize them. Recognize also that these patients frequently vigorously deny their illness - both to their physicians and, sometimes, to themselves.

Without exception, if the patient takes enough drug long enough, he will develop tolerance to it and/or signs of physiological withdrawal when it is stopped; ie, SEDATIVE OR HYPNOTIC DEPENDENCE (DSM-III p 170, 304.1). Some evidence suggests that there is a familial pattern to the abuse of these substances (eg, family members also abuse sedative-hypnotics and alcohol).

SEDATIVE OR HYPNOTIC WITHDRAWAL (DSM-III p 140, 292.00): This is the most dangerous of the drug withdrawal syndromes and can occur both in the dependent person who abstains and also in the person who merely reduces his dose. Its severity depends upon the particular drug abused, the duration of use, and daily dose used (degree of tolerance). Keep a high index of suspicion. Recognize it (1) by a history of significant drug use (often denied by the patient), (2) by characteristic abstinence symptoms (see below), and (3) by a Tolerance Test.

Withdrawal Symptoms:

   Psychological: A subjective sense of severe anxiety, restlessness, apprehension, irritability, insomnia, and anorexia which has developed gradually over the past 24 hours (1-3 days with the longer acting sedative-hypnotics) and is worsening hour by hour. Delirium may occur (SEDATIVE OR HYPNOTIC WITHDRAWAL DELIRIUM, DSM-III p 141, 292.00) with visual hallucinations and formication (sense of insects crawling on the skin).
   Physical: Tremulousness (coarse tremor - primarily the upper extremities), weakness, nausea and vomiting, orthostatic hypotension, tachycardia, hyperreflexia, diaphoresis. After several days this may progress to delirium, hyperpyrexia, and coma. Seizures may occur (typically after 2-5 days) - usually generalized and single or a short series, but occasionally status epilepticus.

Tolerance Test:

There are several methods of determining the degree of dependence (and thus the probable severity and length of withdrawal). One method is given below. It can be used regardless of the particular sedative-hypnotic drug of abuse (ie, they are all cross-tolerant).

1. Hospitalize the patient for the test if possible.
2. Administer test to a patient who is comfortable or only mildly anxious (not to a patient who is intoxicated or presently withdrawing - test would be invalid).
3. Give 200 mg of pentobarbital orally.
4. At one hour, evaluate the patient. If he is:
   a. asleep but arousable - patient has no tolerance.
   b. grossly ataxic, coarse tremor and nystagmus - daily tolerance is 400-500 mg of pentobarbital.
   c. mildly ataxic, mild nystagmus - daily tolerance is 600 mg.
   d. comfortable, slight lateral nystagmus - daily tolerance is 800 mg.
   e. asymptomatic or has continuing signs of mild withdrawal - daily tolerance is 1000 mg, or more. Wait 3-4 hours, then give an oral dose of 300 mg of pentobarbital. Failure to become symptomatic at this larger dose suggests a daily tolerance of greater than 1600 mg.

Treat withdrawal vigorously and carefully. Usually hospitalize unless the addiction is mild and the patient reliable. Evaluate for medical illness. Withdrawal can be accomplished safely using several different sedative-hypnotics although the most commonly used are pentobarbital and phenobarbital.

To withdraw with pentobarbital, give the estimated daily tolerance dose (obtained either by reliable history of all cross-tolerant drugs and alcohol used or by a tolerance test) equally divided on a Q6hr schedule for the first and second days and then reduce 10% of the initial dose each day. Expect the patient to be somewhat uncomfortable but, if signs of serious withdrawal (or intoxication) appear, slow (or quicken) the decrease slightly. If the patient is showing serious withdrawal symptoms before treatment, give enough pentobarbital over several hours to make him comfortable, then begin the withdrawal procedure.

SEDATIVE OR HYPNOTIC AMNESTIC DISORDER (DSM-III p 141, 292.83): This profound, short-term, anterograde and retrograde memory loss (Korsakoff's Syndrome) is usually reversible.

HALLUCINOGENS

DRUGS INVOLVED:

    lysergic acid diethylamide (LSD-25, acid)
    2,5-dimethoxy-4-methylamphetamine (DOM, STP)
    dimethyltryptamine (DMT)
    trimethoxyamphetamine (TMA)
    psilocybin
    mescaline (peyote, tops, cactus)

    phencyclidine (PCP, angel dust, hog)
    thiocyclidine (TCP)
    ketamine (Ketalar)

    cannabis (marijuana, hashish, pot, weed, grass, reefer)
    delta-9-tetrahydrocannabinol (THC)

LSD, MESCALINE, AND OTHERS:

    Patients take these drugs orally, develop symptoms in
10-45 minutes, and are back to normal in several hours (eg,
LSD) to 1-2 days. The typical consequence of ingestion
(HALLUCINOGEN HALLUCINOSIS, DSM-III p 153, 305.30) is:

    Psychological symptoms - Marked perceptual distortions
        (changing object shapes, changing body image),
        illusions, hallucinations (mostly visual geometric
        designs, but also auditory and tactile), depersonal-
        ization, derealization, and synesthesias (stimuli in
        one modality produce sensations in another - eg,
        sounds become colors) - all occurring in a clear
        sensorium. The patient is usually aware that what he
        is experiencing is due to drugs (ie, has insight -
        unlike the patient with amphetamine psychosis).
        Occasionally the patient experiences strong depressive
        or anxious feelings (eg, panic - a "bad trip") but
        more typically the mood is euphoric and the patient
        feels he is receiving profound, staggering insights.
    Physical symptoms - Tachycardia, palpitations, diaphore-
        sis, pupillary dilation (responsive to light), blurred
        vision, tremor, incoordination, hyperreflexia, hyper-
        thermia, piloerection.

The psychological symptoms are particularly sensitive to
the "set" or expectations of the patient prior to drug
usage. Occasionally the patient will experience brief
hallucinations weeks, months, or even years after the
period of drug use (flashbacks). Flashback experiences may
be continued for years, even in the absence of additional
LSD usage, if marijuana is used regularly. Although

primarily used as recreational drugs, a few patients disrupt their lives with drug use (HALLUCINOGEN ABUSE DSM-III p 175, 305.3). There are no withdrawal symptoms although slight tolerance does develop. Two clinical syndromes which may (infrequently) follow the use of these drugs by one or more days are:

HALLUCINOGEN DELUSIONAL DISORDER (DSM-III p 155, 292.11) - Delusions that occur with drug use may persist for a variable length of time after the drug is out of the body.

HALLUCINOGEN AFFECTIVE DISORDER (DSM-III p 156, 292.84) - A persistence of a dysphoric mood (usually depression or anxiety) for days, weeks, or longer after taking the drug. The presentation may be identical to or gradually develop into a major affective disorder.

Treatment for "bad trips" usually consists of support ("talking down") - patient usually clears within hours. Benzodiazepines and phenothiazines may be used (eg, diazepam 10-15 mg; haloperidol 4-5 mg).

PHENCYCLIDINE (PCP):

PCP is an increasingly common drug of abuse PHENCYCLIDINE ABUSE, DSM-III p 174, 305.9), particularly among youth. It is eaten, smoked, or taken IV. Symptoms begin in 2-60 minutes, depending on the route of administration.

Psychological symptoms - Low doses produce euphoria, grandiosity, a feeling of "numbness," and emotional lability. Higher doses cause symptoms which range from perceptual distortions, anxiety, excitation, confusion, and synesthesias to a paranoid psychosis, rigidity, and a catatonic-like state to convulsions, coma, and death. Violent (and self-destructive) behavior is common when intoxicated.
Physical symptoms - Tachycardia, hypertension, vertical and horizontal nystagmus, ataxia, dysarthria, myoclonus, decreased pain sensitivity, diaphoresis, seizures.

The patient usually clears in 3-6 hours. The symptom picture can be quite variable and can include a delirium usually lasting several days but which may last weeks or longer (PHENCYCLIDINE DELIRIUM, DSM-III p 152, 292.81) or a complex and varying presentation of organic features (PHENCYCLIDINE MIXED ORGANIC MENTAL DISEASE, DSM-III p 153, 292.90). Long-term organic symptoms may occur (memory loss, word-finding difficulty). Diagnosis is based on the clinical picture and the presence of PCP in urine.

Treatment is controversial. ODs can be fatal. Hospitalize and use gastric suction, urine acidification, and symptomatic medical maintenance. If agitation must be controlled, use diazepam rather than antipsychotics - also decrease external stimulation.

CANNABIS:

The active ingredient of cannabis is delta-9-tetrahydrocannabinol (THC). The various forms (eg, marijuana, hashish) are all either smoked or eaten and the differences in the effects they produce depend primarily on their concentrations of THC. Cannabis is used widely and usually produces mild physical and psychological alterations (CANNABIS INTOXICATION, DSM-III p 157, 305.20) which occur shortly after intake and last 2-4 hours.

Psychological symptoms - The primary effect is a sense of well-being, mild euphoria, and relaxation. Mild alterations and intensifications of perceptions occur (greater with the more concentrated forms) as does a sense of indifference. A few persons find the use of cannabis dysphoric and develop depression, paranoia, anxiety, or panic. Impaired recent memory during and shortly following use is common (expected).
Physical symptoms - Tachycardia, conjunctival injection, dry mouth, increased appetite.

Toxic psychoses have been reported with high dose use. Some persons are socially and occupationally handicapped by chronic drug use (CANNABIS ABUSE, DSM-III p 175, 305.2). These patients are frequently apathetic and "amotivational" but this may be more a reflection of their personality structure than an effect of cannabis. If there is also a significant degree of tolerance, the patient has CANNABIS DEPENDENCE (DSM-III p 175, 304.3).

Treat "bad trips" with support. Surreptitious use of marijuana can be detected by a urine screen for delta-9-tetrahydrocannabinol-11-oic acid up to 12-24 hours after use (Magliozzi et al, 1983).

STIMULANTS

DRUGS INVOLVED:

amphetamine (Benzedrine)
dextroamphetamine (Dexedrine)

    methamphetamine (Methedrine, "speed")
    phenmetrazine (Preludin)
    cocaine

    These are effective orally (except cocaine), nasally
(cocaine), and by smoking (cocaine) but produce a more
rapid and intense effect IV (an orgasm-like "rush").
Street terms include speed, bennies, uppers, diet pills,
crystal, double crosses, coke or snow (cocaine), and
speedball (amphetamine or cocaine with an opioid).

CLINICAL SYNDROMES:

    The effects of SYMPATHOMIMETIC INTOXICATION (DSM-III p
147, 305.70) and COCAINE INTOXICATION (DSM-III p 145,
305.60) occur within minutes (depending on route) and
consist of:

    Psychological symptoms - Hyperalertness, restlessness,
       psychomotor agitation, pacing, talkativeness and
       pressure of speech, sense of well-being, elation.
       Frequently aggressiveness, violent behavior, and poor
       judgement occur as well.
    Physical symptoms - Tachycardia, hypertension, pupillary
       dilation, chills and diaphoresis, anorexia, nausea and
       vomiting, insomnia. Occasionally there are
       stereotyped repetitive movements (eg, endlessly taking
       something apart and then reassembling it).

With brief use, symptoms usually disappear within hours of
stopping the drug. All these symptoms may disappear as
tolerance develops.

    If drug use becomes a consuming pattern which lasts
for at least one month and which interferes with social and
occupational functioning, the patient has SYMPATHOMIMETIC
ABUSE (DSM-III p 173, 305.7) or COCAINE ABUSE (DSM-III
p 173, 305.6). Abuse usually develops over months and may
include a pattern of "runs" of frequent, large-dose IV
administration over days or weeks. After a run, the person
frequently sleeps for 12-18 hours, then may begin another
run. High dose use places the patient at risk for
developing:

    SYMPATHOMIMETIC DEPENDENCE (DSM-III p 173, 304.4) - ie,
       tolerance and/or withdrawal present.

    SYMPATHOMIMETIC DELIRIUM (DSM-III p 148, 292.81) - A
       characteristic organic delirium (see chapter 5)
       develops shortly after taking the drug and disappears
       as the blood level drops. Violence is common during
       these episodes.

SYMPATHOMIMETIC DELUSIONAL DISORDER (DSM-III p 149,
292.11) - Patient becomes markedly paranoid and
develops persecutory delusions within a setting of
clear consciousness, often accompanied by hostility,
anxiety, ideas of reference, and psychomotor agitation.
This condition may last for one week or longer than
one year. It easily can be mistaken for paranoid
schizophrenia, which it closely resembles.

SYMPATHOMIMETIC WITHDRAWAL (DSM-III p 150, 292.00) -
Cessation of drug in heavy user may be followed by
mild to severe depression (watch for suicide), profound
fatigue, irritability, anxiety, fearfulness, nightmares,
and insomnia or hypersomnia. Severe symptoms seldom
last more than one week but may be followed by chronic
low-level depression and/or anxiety. Abnormal EEG
patterns may last for weeks.

Make the diagnosis by the clinical picture and history
of drug use. Most sympathomimetics and cocaine can be
identified by a urine drug screen (cocaine is difficult -
check with your lab).

TREATMENT:

Stop the drug. If the patient is mildly or moderately
excited - try to "talk him down" and use benzodiazepines.
The patient may be agitated and violent - take appropriate
precautions (eg, restraints). Treat severe intoxication,
delirium, and delusional symptoms with an antipsychotic
(eg, haloperidol 5-10 mg PO or 5 mg IM). Acidify the urine
with ascorbic acid or ammonium chloride (maintain Ph at 4-
5). Be alert to potential suicide and to medical complications (eg, MI, stroke, intracranial hemorrhage). Severe
withdrawal depressions may respond to antidepressants.

INHALANTS

The types of glues, solvents, and cleaners "sniffed"
for their psychic effects are numerous and include gasoline,
kerosene, plastic and rubber cements, airplane and
household glues, paints, lacquers, enamels, paint thinners,
solvents, aerosols, furniture polishes, fingernail polish
removers, nitrous oxide, cleaning fluids, etc. Several
active constituents are probably involved in most
substances. This is a major abuse problem, particularly
among late latency and early to middle adolescent children,
and particularly among lower socioeconomic groups. This is
often a group activity.

The effects from this variety of substances are usually quite similar - typically mild euphoria, confusion, disorientation, impulsivity, and ataxia - all of which may progress to a toxic psychosis, seizures, and coma. Repeated and chronic abuse is common but withdrawal symptoms have not been noticed. Death has occurred from asphyxiation, aspiration, cardiac arrhythmias, and kidney, liver, and bone marrow damage. An acute brain syndrome (delirium) typically occurs but only in the unusual or very severe case does the patient appear to develop a degree of chronic CNS damage.

Physical restraint and medical support may be needed in the acute situation but the patient usually clears over hours or days. Evaluate carefully for liver, kidney, and pulmonary damage. Encourage these children and their families to enter therapy.

REFERENCES

1. Abraham HD: Visual phenomenology of the LSD flashback. Arch Gen Psychiat 40:884, 1983.
2. Aronow R, Done AK: Phencyclidine overdose: an emerging concept of management. J Am Coll Emerg Physician 7:56, 1978.
3. Bergman H, Borg S, Holm L: Neuropsychological impairment and exclusive abuse of sedatives or hypnotics. Am J Psychiat 137:215, 1980.
4. Charney DS, Riordan CE, Kleber HD, Murburg M, Braverman P, Sternberg DE, Heninger GR, Redmond E: Clonidine and naltrexone. Arch Gen Psychiat 39:1327, 1982.
5. Connell LJ, Berlin RM: Withdrawal after substitution of a short-acting for a long-acting benzodiazepine. JAMA 250:2838, 1983.
6. Domino EF: PCP (Phencyclidine): Historical and Current Perspectives. Ann Arbor, MI, NPP Books, 1981.
7. Gold MS, Pottash AC, Sweeney DR, Kleber HD: Opiate withdrawal using clonidine. JAMA 243:343, 1980.
8. Hofmann FG: A Handbook on Drug and Alcohol Abuse: The Biomedical Aspects. New York, Oxford Univ Pr, 1975.
9. Judson BA, Goldstein A, Inturrisi CE: Methadyl acetate (LAAM) in the treatment of heroin addicts. Arch Gen Psychiat 40:834, 1983.
10. Leung FW, Guze PA: Diazepam withdrawal. West J Med 138:96, 1983.
11. Magliozzi JR, Kanter SL, Csernansky JG, Hollister LE: Detection of marajuana use in psychiatric patients by determination of urinary delta-9-tetrahydrocannabinol-11-oic acid. J Nerv Ment Dis 171:246, 1983.

12. Rounsaville BJ, Weissman MM, Kleber H, Wilber C: Heterogeneity of psychiatric diagnosis in treated opiate addicts. Arch Gen Psychiat 39:161, 1982.
13. Sato M, Chen C, Akiyama I, Otsuki S: Acute exacerbation of paranoid psychotic state after long-term abstinence in patients with previous methamphetamine psychosis. Biol Psychiat 18:429, 1983.
14. Weller RA, Halikas JA: Objective criteria for the diagnosis of marijuana abuse. J Nerv Ment Dis 168:98, 1980.
15. Winokur A, Rickels K, Greenblatt DJ, Snyder PJ, Schatz NJ: Withdrawal reaction from long-term low-dosage administration of diazepam. Arch Gen Psychiat 37:101, 1980.
16. Woody GE, Luborsky L, McLellan AT, O'Brien CP, Beck AT, Blaine J, Herman I, Hole A: Psychotherapy for opiate addicts. Arch Gen Psychiat 40:639, 1983.

Chapter 18

Personality Disorders

Personality is a consistent style of behavior uniquely recognizable in each individual. Personality disorders (Axis II of DSM-III) refers to personality characteristics of a form or magnitude that are maladaptive and which cause poor life functioning. These long-term traits feel "natural" (ego syntonic) even though a person may be bothered by the results of his behavior. There are elements of the personality disorders in all of us and the difference between health and pathology may be one of degree. Moreover, many patients display their pathology clearly only when under stress.

Most personality disorders develop in childhood and become fixed by the early 20's yet some occur following organic insults to the brain. Some may have a biologic, and even a genetic, component (eg, Antisocial Personality Disorder). Psychological testing may facilitate diagnosis: WAIS, MMPI, Bender Gestalt, and Rorschach. Atypical and mixed types are common and some may grade into or be confused with similar psychoses (eg, paranoid type : Paranoid Schizophrenia). These patients often resist treatment and change slowly, but occasionally respond to a variety of treatment modalities including individual or group therapy, and short term use of antianxiety agents or low doses of major tranquilizers. Some may require inpatient treatment during periods of decompensation. Adolescents (under 18), and even children, may receive a personality disorder diagnosis if the pattern is stable, clear, and incompatible with a childhood disorder.

ANTISOCIAL P.D. (DSM-III p 317, 301.70)

The antisocial behavior invariably begins in childhood or early adolescence: aggressiveness, fighting, "hyperactivity," poor peer relationships, irresponsibility, lying, theft, truancy, poor school performance, runaway, inappropriate sexual activity, drug and alcohol use. As adults there is criminality, assaultiveness, self-defeating

impulsivity, hedonism, promiscuity, unreliability, and
crippling drug and alcohol abuse. They fail at work,
change jobs frequently, go AWOL and receive dishonorable
discharges from the service, are abusing parents and
neglectful mates, can't maintain intimate interpersonal
relationships, and spend time in jails and prisons. These
patients are frequently, if temporarily, anxious and
depressed (suicide gestures) and are second only to
patients with hysteria in the production of conversion
symptoms. The behavior peaks in late adolescence and the
early 20's with improvement in the 30's although the
patients rarely recover from the "lost years." Males are
involved more severely, earlier, and more frequently (3% of
population) - M:F = 5-10:1.

Their rearing is generally impaired by rejection,
neglect, desertion, poverty, and inconsistent discipline -
they are frequently illegitimate and unwanted. The parents
are often criminals (30% of fathers), alcoholics (50% of
fathers), and chronically unemployed. Male first degree
relatives have an increased incidence of Antisocial
Personality Disorder, alcoholism, and drug abuse and female
relatives have associated Briquet's Syndrome. A genetic
component is likely (Cadoret, 1978).

No tests are diagnostic although a 4-9 MMPI profile is
common and there is an increased incidence of non-specific
EEG abnormalities (increased slow-wave activity, etc). It
is necessary to rule out primary drug and alcohol abuse
(difficult, look for normal childhood behavior),
schizophrenia (thought disorder present), OBS
(disorientation, memory impairment), early mania, explosive
disorder, and ADULT ANTISOCIAL BEHAVIOR (DSM-III p 332,
V71.01). Several very specialized disorders of impulse
control can also mimic this disorder: PATHOLOGICAL GAMBLING
(DSM-III p 291, 312.31), KLEPTOMANIA (DSM-III p 293,
312.32), and PYROMANIA (DSM-III p 294, 312.33). The
patients are resistant and manipulative - don't rely on the
patient's report; check your data. They rarely seek help
for personality change and treatment is difficult and often
unsuccessful. Best results follow closely supervised
inpatient care: utilize strong, frequent, and accurate
confrontation of interpersonal behavior, particularly by
peers. Individual outpatient psychotherapy is of little
value. The terms antisocial personality disorder,
sociopathy, and psychopathy generally are used synonymously.

HISTRIONIC P.D. (DSM-III p 313, 301.50)

Histrionic patients initially seem charming, likeable,
lively, and seductive but gradually become seen as

emotionally unstable, egocentric, immature, dependant, manipulative, excitement-seeking, and shallow. They demand attention, are exhibitionistic, and present a "caricature of femininity" yet have a limited ability to maintain stable, intimate interpersonal relationships with either sex. This common disorder occurs predominantly in women. There is an association with depression, transient psychoses, substance abuse, and Conversion and (particularly) Somatization Disorders. Suicidal gestures and attempts are common. Lesser impaired patients respond to psychotherapy.

BORDERLINE P.D. (DSM-III P 321, 301.83)

These usually socially adapted patients have complex clinical presentations including diverse combinations of anger, anxiety, intense and labile affect, brief disturbances in consciousness (eg, depersonalization, dissociation), chronic loneliness, boredom, a chronic sense of emptiness, volatile interpersonal relations, identity confusion, and impulsive behavior including self-injury. Stress can precipitate a transient psychosis. Many other diagnoses are often suggested or can also be made; eg, depression, Brief Reactive Psychosis, other personality disorders, Cyclothymic Disorder. This is a heterogeneous group, some of whom may be related genetically to schizophrenia or affective disorders (Loranger et al, 1982). Psychological testing is useful. Be sure to rule out organic states such as mild delirium, psychomotor epilepsy, or use of LSD. Insight oriented and supportive psychotherapies (and their combination) are often beneficial. Low-dose antipsychotic agents (thioridazine 100-300 mg hs), antidepressants, or lithium carbonate may help selected patients.

NARCISSISTIC P.D. (DSM-III p 315, 301.81)

Although often symptom-free and well functioning, these patients are chronically dissatisfied due to a constant need for admiration and habitually unrealistic self-expectations. They are impulsive and anxious, have ideas of omnipotence and of being a "special person," become quickly dissatisfied with others, and maintain superficial, exploitative interpersonal relationships. Under stress and when their needs are not met, they may become depressed, develop somatic complaints, have brief psychotic episodes, or display extreme rage. Mixtures with other personality disorders are common. Long-term psychotherapy helps.

PASSIVE-AGGRESSIVE P.D. (DSM-III p 328, 301.84)

These patients are irritating and infuriating. They are oppositional, resentful, and controlling and thus have few friends and significantly impaired social and occupational functioning. Their enormous hostility is expressed passively - by intentional inefficiency, negativism, stubborness, procrastination, "forgetfulness," withdrawal, and somatic complaints. They are overdependent on other people and institutions yet resist demands made on them, even if able to perform. This disorder is common, stable over time, and associated with episodes of anxiety and depression as well as alcoholism, drug dependency, and an "inability to cope." Long-term individual psychotherapy may be useful.

PARANOID P.D. (DSM-III p 307, 301.00)

These aloof, emotionally cold people typically display unjustified suspiciousness, hypersensitivity to slights, jealousy, and a fear of intimacy. They tend to be grandiose, rigid, contentious, and litigious and are thus isolated and disliked. They accept criticism poorly, blaming others instead. This disorder may be associated with chronic CNS impairment, drug use (eg, amphetamines), and obsessive-compulsive states. Psychotic decompensation sometimes occurs, requiring major tranquilizers. They rarely seek treatment.

SCHIZOID P.D. (DSM-III p 310, 301.20)

These are seclusive people who have little wish or capacity to form interpersonal relations, derive little pleasure from social contacts, and yet can perform well if left alone (eg, night watchman). They have a limited emotional range, daydream excessively, and are humorless and aloof. They do not appear to have an increased risk of developing schizophrenia as was previously thought (Parnas et al, 1982). Treatment seems of little help.

SCHIZOTYPAL P.D. (DSM-III p 312, 301.22)

In addition to having features of the schizoid, these people are "peculiar." They relate strange intrapsychic experiences, reason in odd ways, and are difficult to "get to know" yet none of these features reach psychotic proportions. Schizophrenia occurs with increased frequency in family members (Baron et al, 1983), suggesting that this condition is part of the "schizophrenic spectrum" of disorders.

COMPULSIVE P.D. (DSM-III p 326, 301.40)

These patients, frequently successful men, are inhibited, stubborn, perfectionistic, judgmental, overly conscientious, rigid, and chronically anxious individuals who avoid intimacy and experience little pleasure from life. They are indecisive yet demanding and are often perceived as cold and reserved. They are at risk to develop Obsessive Compulsive Disorder and depression. Psychotherapy can effect changes over time.

AVOIDANT P.D. (DSM-III p 323, 301.82)

This is a fairly common disorder: an exceedingly shy, lonely, hypersensitive individual with low self-esteem who would rather avoid personal contact than face any potential social disapproval, even though desperate for interpersonal involvement (as opposed to the schizoid person). These patients are troubled by anxiety and depression.

DEPENDENT P.D. (DSM-III p 324, 301.60)

These are excessively passive, unsure, isolated people who become abnormally dependent on one or more people. Initially acceptable, the behavior can become very controlling, appear hostile, and blend into a passive-aggressive style. It is more common in women and is likely to lead to anxiety and depression, particularly if the dependent relationship is threatened.

ATTENTION DEFICIT DISORDER, RESIDUAL TYPE (DSM-III p 44, 314.80) is a disorder of children which continues to produce problems well into adulthood and which has many features of a personality disorder. These patients have been distractible, impulsive, quick tempered, unable to tolerate stress, and restless since childhood (Wender et al, 1981). Their lability impairs interpersonal relations and job stability and results in frequent depressions. They are at risk for drug abuse and alcoholism (Wood et al, 1983). Differentiate from personality disorders, Cyclothymic Disorder (more recent onset), Intermittent Explosive Disorder (normal between episodes), and primary depression. ADD is most effectively treated with stimulants (eg, methylphenidate 10mg PO TID) but use them very cautiously due to abuse potential. Combine with supportive psychotherapy.

REFERENCES

1. Akhtar S, Thomson JA: Overview: Narcissistic Personality Disorder. Am J Psychiat 139:12, 1982.
2. Baron M, Gruen R, Asnis L, Kane J: Familial relatedness of schizophrenia and schizotypal states. Am J Psychiat 140:1437, 1983.
3. Bohman M, Cloninger CR, Sigvardsson S, von Knorring A: Predisposition to petty criminality in Swedish adoptees. Arch Gen Psychiat 39:1233, 1982.
4. Cadoret RJ: Psychopathology in adopted-away offspring of biologic parents with antisocial behavior. Arch Gen Psychiat 35:176, 1978.
5. Chodoff P: Hysteria and women. Am J Psychiat 139:545, 1982.
6. Frosh JP: Current Perspectives on Personality Disorders. APA Press, Washington, DC, 1983.
7. Lion JR: Personality Disorders. Williams & Wilkins Co, Baltimore, 1981.
8. Loranger AW, Oldham JM, Tulis EH: Familial transmission of DSM-III borderline personality disorder. Arch Gen Psychiat 39:795, 1982.
9. Millon TM: Disorders of Personality. John Wiley & Sons, New York, 1981.
10. Nurnberg HG, Suh R: Time-limited psychotherapy of the hospitalized borderline patient. Amer J Psychotherapy 37:82, 1982.
11. Parnas J, Schulsinger F, Schulsinger H, Mednick SA, Teasdale TW: Behavioral precursors of schizophrenic spectrum. Arch Gen Psychiat 39:658, 1982.
12. Pollak, JM: Obsessive-compulsive personality: a review. Psycho Bull 86:225, 1979.
13. Pope HG, Jonas JM, Hudson JI, Cohen BM, Gunderson JG: The validity of DSM-III borderline personality disorder. Arch Gen Psychiat 40:23, 1983.
14. Small IF, Small JG, Alig VB, Moore DF: Passive-aggressive personality disorder: a search for a syndrome. Am J Psychiat 126:973, 1970.
15. Wender PH, Reimherr FW, Wood DR: Attention deficit disorder ("minimal brain dysfunction") in adults: a replication study of diagnosis and drug treatment. Arch Gen Psychiat 38:449, 1981.
16. Wood DR, Wender PH, Reimherr FW: The prevalence of attention deficit disorder, residual type, or minimal brain dysfunction, in a population of male alcoholic patients. Am J Psychiat 140:95, 1983.

Chapter 19

Psychosexual Disorders

These disorders are often first brought to the attention of the general physician. The three distinct categories are:

Psychosexual Dysfunction - inhibition in sexual desire and/ or psychophysiological performance.
Paraphilia - sexual arousal to deviant stimuli.
Gender Identity Disorders - patient feels like the opposite sex.

PSYCHOSEXUAL DYSFUNCTION

Clinically observable features of the normal human sexual response cycle consist of (Masters and Johnson, 1966):

Stage I: Excitement (minutes to hours)
  males - psychological arousal and penile erection.
  females - psychological arousal, vaginal lubrication, nipple erection, and vasocongestion of the external genitalia.

Stage II: Plateau (seconds to 3 minutes)
  males - several drops of fluid appear at head of penis (from Cowper's gland).
  females - tightening of outer third of vagina, breast engorgement.

Stage III: Orgasm (5-15 seconds)
  males - ejaculation, involuntary muscular contraction (eg, pelvis); followed by a refractory period.
  females - contractions of outer third of vagina, some involuntary pelvic thrusting; may be multiple.

Stage IV: Resolution
  males - relaxation, detumescence, sense of well-being.
  females - relaxation, detumescence, sense of well-being.

Patients (or their partners) may complain of decreased sexual desire and/or of one or more specific abnormalities of the response cycle. The dysfunctions may be situational, partial rather than complete, and primary or acquired. The phases usually occur in a stepwise fashion but that is not mandatory - identify the stage involved. Often there are marital problems, unrealistic expectations, long-standing personal "hangups", chronic difficulty establishing and maintaining intimate interpersonal relations, etc. Identify these through history and psychiatric evaluation. Always evaluate carefully for organic causes (particularly with impotence and dyspareunia). Organic conditions tend to be chronic and independent of the situation.

Treatment should be global with an emphasis on intimacy and relationship - not just technique. Identify and treat psychosocial causes with dynamic psychotherapy, marital therapy, hypnotherapy, and group therapy. Sedatives may help temporarily if anxiety is prominent. Even purely physical causes often have significant associated secondary interpersonal problems that must be addressed once the medical condition has been corrected. A good prognosis is associated with acute, recent dysfunction in a psychologically healthy patient with good past sexual functioning and strong sexual interests. Some relationships between partners are sufficiently hostile and destructive that, unless other matters are resolved, prognosis is very poor for a correction of the psychosexual dysfunction.

The "new sex therapy" (Masters and Johnson, 1970) uses individual psychotherapy, couples therapy, education, behavior modification techniques, and often a male-female therapist pair (dual-sex therapy). Their numerous techniques have wide applicability with sexual dysfunctions and should be considered for use. Many of these methods center on decreasing a patient's (or couple's) anxiety about making love. Essential principles include:

- Good communication with full exploration of sexual feelings
- Training in specific stimulation and coital techniques (through "pleasuring sessions")
- Emphasis on the couple as a pleasure-giving team
- Prohibition of intercourse early in therapy (to reduce performance anxiety)
- Emphasis on multi-modal sensory pleasure (touch, sight, sound) and sensory awareness exercises
- Insistence that physiological responses be ignored (erection, etc. - "don't worry about it; it will happen")

INHIBITED SEXUAL EXCITEMENT (DSM-III p 279, 3O2.72):

Males (impotence): The failure to reach or maintain a
complete erection in at least 75% of attempts. Two forms
exist:

Primary impotence - Patient has never maintained an
    erection.
Secondary impotence - Patient has lost the ability. This
    may be person or situation specific (selective
    impotence).

Impotence is the most common sexual complaint of men -
predominantly the secondary form. It is not a "natural
consequence" of aging.

Some feel 90% of cases are psychogenic but recent
studies (Spark, 1980; Karacan, 1982) emphasize the
frequency of an organic etiology. Organic causes include:

- Disorders of the hypothalamic-pituitary-gonadal axis: Low
    serum testosterone level due to primary testicular
    hypofunction, pituitary tumors, etc.
- Endocrine: Hyperthyroidism (may have elevated testos-
    terone), hyperprolactinemia, diabetes mellitus,
    acromegaly, Addison's disease, myxedema.
- Medication: Tricyclic antidepressants, MAOIs, major
    tranquilizers (particularly thioridazine), cholinergic
    blockers, antihypertensive drugs (particularly
    adrenergic blockers and false sympathetic neuro-
    transmitters), estrogens, ethyl alcohol (alcoholism),
    addictive drugs (particularly narcotics and ampheta-
    mines), anticholinergic drugs.
- Illness: Any illness may cause impotence temporarily but
    particularly chronic debilitating disease, chronic
    renal disease, peripheral vascular disease, and local
    physical and neurological disorders.

Psychogenic causes include depression, anxiety (over
cardiac status, performance, etc.), hostility and marital
conflict, etc.

First identify any physical cause - do a complete
medical evaluation (look for physical illness, absent beard
and body hair, small testes, gynecomastia), get serum
testosterone (then further hormonal studies if low). Early
morning sleeping erection or occasional successful
intercourse does not rule out an organic etiology nor does
a normal pattern of nocturnal penile tumescence (NPT -
erections during REM sleep) rule in a psychogenic etiology,
although most (all?) psychogenic cases have normal NPT.

Treat medical causes (often curative). Follow with global
therapy, if needed. Therapy includes allowing the female
to play the dominant role and insisting on a gradual shift
from foreplay to intercourse. Perhaps 30-40% will not
improve.

Females (frigidity): An inadequate genital sexual response
(failure to reach the excitement or plateau stages)
although the woman may find sexual activity pleasurable.
It often reflects personality or marital problems but other
specific causes include poor physical health, alcoholism,
fatigue, depression, fear of pregnancy, and a postpartum
state. Treat the couple.

PREMATURE EJACULATION (DSM-III p 280, 302.75):

The ejaculation occurs before the patient wishes it to
(usually before his partner reaches orgasm). 40% of all
patients with sexual complaints. Cause is usually
functional and secondary to anxiety (determine the source
of the anxiety). It is much more common in stressful
marriages. "Squeeze technique" effective - just prior to
ejaculation, woman squeezes head of glans. This is coupled
with the man practicing imagery control. The young and
vigorous male may benefit from 1% Nupercaine ointment
applied to the coronal ridge and frenulum.

INHIBITED MALE ORGASM (DSM-III p 280, 302.74):
(Retarded Ejaculation)

The patient fails to ejaculate. Differentiate from
retrograde ejaculation ("ejaculation" into the bladder -
due to organic factors; eg, anticholinergic drugs,
prostatectomy). Some patients can have an orgasm only
under certain conditions (eg, with masturbation, with a
stranger) - identify the circumstances in which orgasm can
take place. Psychological causes include lack of interest
(eg, primary sexual deviation), anxiety, compulsive
personality, marriage stresses, and sexual "hangups."
Physical causes include medication (guanethidine,
methyldopa, phenothiazines - particularly thioridazine,
MAOIs), GU surgery, and lower spinal cord impairment (eg,
parkinsonism, syringomyelia). First train the patient to
ejaculate by himself, then treat the interpersonal
relationship - individual psychotherapy is often needed.
The technique of the female self-inserting her partner's
penis may be effective.

INHIBITED FEMALE ORGASM (DSM-III p 279, 302.73)
(Anorgasmia):

The patient persistently fails to reach orgasm during intercourse. There are primary (5% of cases) and secondary forms although be aware that many women become orgasmic as they get older (peak at age 35). There may be a hormonal basis in some but most causes are psychological. This condition is very situation specific - some women never have orgasm in spite of ample excitement (10%), others have orgasm only with masturbation, still others require clitoral manipulation during intercourse, and a minority of women can have an orgasm with intercourse alone. Psychotherapy involves first training the woman to have an orgasm by herself, then treating the couple.

FUNCTIONAL DYSPAREUNIA (DSM-III p 280, 302.76):

Pain with intercourse. It often is related to a physical condition (50%): cervical or vaginal infection or anatomic abnormality, endometriosis, tumor, or other pelvic pathology. Anxiety about sexual activity (for a variety of reasons) can produce pelvic muscle tightening and pain but, remember, pain from organic causes can produce anxiety which exacerbates the pain. Also, dyspareunia can produce vaginismus and vaginismus can produce dyspareunia.

FUNCTIONAL VAGINISMUS (DSM-III p 280, 306.51):

The patient has an involuntary spasm during coitus of the muscles surrounding the outer third of the vagina which prevents penile entrance. It may be related to physical causes producing pain - dyspareunia. Psychological causes include past sexual trauma (eg, rape), a hostile marital relationship (perhaps from a vicious cycle), or sexual "hangups." Individual therapy and relaxation techniques are usually required. Hegar dilators (size increased over 3-5 days) may be useful.

INHIBITED SEXUAL DESIRE (DSM-III p 278, 302.71):

Common and difficult to treat. It may present as inhibited excitement or inhibited orgasm - don't be misled. Causes usually are functional. It varies with time, the sexual partner, depression, anxiety, and the stresses of the relationship. It may reflect a fear of intimacy or pregnancy, a passive-aggressive personality style, strong religious orthodoxy, or homosexuality, among others. Individual or couple therapy is useful.

PARAPHILIA (Sexual Deviation)

These patients become sexually excited only by unusual or bizarre stimuli (practices or fantasies). The particular type of arousing stimulus determines the diagnosis. Orgastic release usually occurs by masturbation during or following the event. Etiology is uncertain - possibly biological, learned, and/or dynamic-instinctual. Most types are rare (courts see them most frequently) although physicians will occasionally encounter them. Men predominate although women may display sadomasochism, voyeurism, and homosexuality.

These patients may not be troubled by their desires (ego-syntonic) and thus are difficult to treat although depression, anxiety, and guilt does occasionally occur. These conditions frequently coexist with personality disorders, alcohol and drug abuse, and other psychiatric disorders - treat them. The patients often have impaired interpersonal relationships, particularly heterosexual relations.

Psychotherapy is frequently unsuccessful. Specific behavior modification techniques to eliminate the deviation are most successful (eg, aversion - covert conditioning) although these must be paired with a more global retraining program (Barlow, 1974). Hypersexual states and some other sexual deviations may benefit from medroxyprogesterone acetate (Depo-Provera) or cyproterone acetate (Berlin and Meinecke, 1981).

PEDOPHILIA (DSM-III p 271, 302.20):

These patients repeatedly approach prepubertal children sexually (touch, explore, mutually masturbate; occasionally intercourse). They are usually timid, inadequate males who know the child involved (a neighbor, relative). Three general types are recognized: heterosexual pedophilia (prefers preadolescent girls), homosexual pedophilia (prefers early teenage boys - most resistant to therapy), and mixed pedophilia (younger children, either sex). Don't confuse with child molestation due to decreased impulse control (eg, OBS, intoxication, retardation, psychosis) or a one-time event (eg, due to loneliness or following a marital crisis). Behavior modification is the treatment of choice.

EXHIBITIONISM (DSM-III p 272, 302.40):

Usually timid males who become sexually aroused by exposing their genitals to an unsuspecting female (adult or child). Only rarely aggressive. Often masturbates during the exposure and needs a shock reaction from the female for satisfaction. Very resistant to treatment.

Less frequent paraphilias include:

   FETISHISM (DSM-III p 268, 302.81): Sexual arousal to
      inanimate objects. May be combined with other sexual
      preferences.
   TRANSVESTISM (DSM-III p 269, 302.30): Aroused by female
      clothing and cross-dressing. Don't confuse with
      transsexualism (the wish to become a female) or
      effeminate homosexuality (cross-dressing is to attract
      others - not to produce arousal itself).
   ZOOPHILIA (DSM-III p 270, 302.10): Sexual activity
      and/or intercourse with animals is the preferred
      method of sexual arousal.
   VOYEURISM (DSM-III p 272, 302.82): Sexual arousal by
      watching unsuspecting people who are naked or sexually
      active. Masturbation usually takes place concurrently.
   SEXUAL SADISM (DSM-III p 274, 302.84): Sexual excitement
      following inflicting psychological or physical (sexual
      or nonsexual) harm on a consenting or nonconsenting
      partner. Some rapists deserve this diagnosis.

                    GENDER IDENTITY DISORDER

TRANSSEXUALISM (DSM-III p 261, 302.5):

     These adults have experienced at least two continuous
years of discomfort about their anatomic sex and have a
desire to change their sex. Males are more common and
their clinical characteristics are more variable. They may
have experienced the discomfort since childhood or only
recently. They may be homosexual, heterosexual, or have
little sexual interest. Many have an effeminate appearance
and cross-dress. Females with this disorder are usually
homosexual and masculine appearing.

     Etiology is unclear - it may be predominantly
biological and/or psychological, although the mother/child
bond always appears disturbed (often too close). Check
karyotype and sex hormone levels. These patients are very
likely to have personality disorders, particularly of the
borderline type. The course is chronic and there is
significant risk for depression, suicide, anxiety, and
genital self-mutilation. Rule out effeminate homosexuality
(patient does not want to be the other sex), schizophrenia,
and hermaphroditism.

Treat with supportive psychotherapy and feminizing/ masculinizing hormones. Sex change surgery (castration, penectomy, vaginoplasty, phalloplasty) is falling out of fashion. It is irreversible and the results appear no better (perhaps worse) than psychotherapy alone. There have been isolated reports of gender identity changes with intensive behavior modification (Barlow et al, 1979).

HOMOSEXUALITY

Homosexuality (an arousal to and preference for sexual relations with adults of the same sex) is not currently considered to be a mental disorder, except if the patient is chronically distressed by it. It may be a temporary phase during adolescence.

Homosexuality is common in the USA - 5-10% of males and perhaps 2-4% of females. In spite of numerous theoretical explanations, the cause(s) is unknown. There may be congenital, prenatal, and/or biological etiologies for some but environmental factors probably dominate in the choice of a sexual orientation.

EGO-DYSTONIC HOMOSEXUALITY (DSM-III p 281, 302.00):

These patients have internalized a negative attitude toward homosexual behavior and chronically and consistently want to change. They suffer from depression, anxiety, and shame.

Most psychotherapy is of little value. However, specialized behavior modification techniques (concentrating on decreasing deviant arousal, stimulating heterosexual arousal, and teaching heterosocial skills) may help as many as 50% (Barlow, 1974).

REFERENCES

1. Barlow DH: The treatment of sexual deviation: toward a comprehensive behavioral approach, in Calhoun K, Adams H, Mitchell K: Innovative Treatment Methods in Psychopathology. New York, John Wiley & Son, 1974.
2. Barlow DH, Abel GG, Blanchard EB: Gender identity change in transsexuals. Arch Gen Psychiat 36:1001, 1979.
3. Berlin FS, Meinecke CF: Treatment of sex offenders with antiandrogenic medication. Am J Psychiat 138:601, 1981.
4. Beutler LE, Gleason DM: Integrating the advances in the diagnosis and treatment of male potency disturbance. J Urol 126:336, 1981.

5. Chalkley AJ, Powell GE: A clinical description of fourty-eight cases of sexual fetishism. Brit J Psychiat 142:292, 1983.
6. Heiman JR, LoPiccolo J: Clinical outcome of sex therapy. Arch Gen Psychiat 40:443, 1983.
7. Hunt DD, Hampson JL: Follow-up of 17 biologic male transsexuals after sex-reassignment surgery. Am J Psychiat 137:432, 1980.
8. Kaplan HS: The New Sex Therapy. New York, Brunner/Mazel, 1974.
9. Karacan I: Nocturnal penile tumescence as a biological marker in assessing erectile dysfunction. Psychosomatics 23:349, 1982.
10. Lothstein LM: Sex reassignment surgery: historical, bioethical, and theoretical issues. Am J Psychiat 139:417, 1982.
11. Masters WH, Johnson VE: Human Sexual Response. Boston, Little, Brown & Co, 1966.
12. Masters WH, Johnson VE: Human Sexual Inadequacy. Boston, Little, Brown & Co, 1970.
13. Saghir MR, Robins E: Male and Female Homosexuality. Baltimore, Williams & Wilkins, 1973.
14. Schover LR, Friedman JM, Weiler SJ, Heiman JR, LoPiccolo J: Multiaxial problem-oriented system for sexual dysfunctions. Arch Gen Psychiat 39:614, 1982.
15. Spark RF, White RA, Connolly PB: Impotence is not always psychogenic. JAMA 243:750, 1980.
16. Symposium on sexual dysfunction. Brit J Psychiat 140:69, 1982.
17. Wasserman MD, Pollak CP, Spielman AJ, Weitzman EO: The differential diagnosis of impotence. JAMA 243:2038, 1980.

Chapter 20

Sleep Disturbances

Sleep disorders are extremely common - 10-20% of the population has had trouble sleeping within the past year; 3-4% have hypersomnia.

Current classification and understanding of sleep problems rests on recent advances in knowledge of normal sleep. Much of this has been obtained through physiological (sleep EEG, EMG, etc) measures of patients in sleep laboratories.

NORMAL SLEEP

Normal sleep is cyclical (4-5 cycles/night) and active, not passive. Distinct stages (measured by EEG) occur and a person passes stepwise through them. Patients enter stage 1, descend by steps over approximately 30 minutes to stage 4, plateau there for 30-40 minutes, and then ascend to lighter stages (1-2) in order to enter REM sleep 90-100 minutes after falling asleep. Then the cycle repeats. As the night progresses, the REM periods lengthen, stage 4 disappears, and the sleep is generally lighter. The length of time spent in any one stage varies in a characteristic fashion with age. The significance of each stage is not known.

Waking - alpha waves (8-12 cps)

NREM Sleep (Non-rapid eye movement) - low level of activity: lowered BP, heart rate, temperature, and respiratory rate. Good muscle tone and slow, drifting eye movements.

Stage 1 - lightest sleep, a transition stage; low voltage, desynchronized waves.
Stage 2 - sleep spindles (13-15 cps) and high spikes (K complexes).

Stage 3 - some delta waves (high voltage at 0.5-2.5
   cps).
Stage 4 - deepest sleep, mostly in first half of
   night; mostly delta waves.

REM Sleep - active sleep characterized by rapid
   synchronous eye movements, twitching of facial and
   extremity muscles, penile erections, and variation in
   pulse, BP, and respiratory rate. Muscular paralysis
   (absent tone) is present. Depth is similar to stage 2.
   Dreaming can occur in several stages but is most
   common in REM sleep.

For clinical purposes, patients with sleep disorders
can be divided into those presenting with complaints of
insomnia or hypersomnia. In each category, there are
several distinct syndromes which must be ruled out.

INSOMNIA

Sleep laboratory studies usually are not needed for
diagnosis and treatment. Take a good history of the sleep
problem, including the 24-hour sleep-wake cycle. Identify
the pattern: trouble falling asleep, trouble staying asleep
(frequent awakenings), early morning awakenings. Inquire
about life stresses, drug and alcohol use, marital and
family problems. Consider the following:

- Is the insomnia simply normal sleep?
   a. Some "insomniacs" get ample sleep (pseudoinsomnia).
      The problems are psychological and lie elsewhere -
      use psychotherapy and reassurance about the adequacy
      of the sleep.
   b. Sleep time lessens with age - explain to concerned
      elderly. Help them avoid a complicating "worry over
      sleeplessness" cycle.
   c. Some patients are substance abusers seeking drugs.

- Is the insomnia transient (situational insomnia)?
   Patient usually has trouble falling asleep. Identify
   the stress. Help the patient correct and deal with it.
   Consider time-limited (1-2 weeks) use of sleeping
   medication (eg, flurazepam, 15-30 mg, PO, HS; triazolam,
   0.25-0.5 mg, PO, HS).

-Is there a chronic, minor psychiatric illness?
   Insomnia is due most frequently to chronic depression
   and/or anxiety. Antisocial and obsessive-compulsive
   features are also common among these patients. They
   often self-medicate, producing more insomnia.

Insomniacs often have trouble expressing aggressive feelings, internalize their problems, and/or have a fear of losing control. The resulting problem is usually sleep onset in type with decreased stage 4 sleep. These patients must be differentiated from those with conditioned insomnia, in which the patient has inadvertently trained himself to stay awake at bedtime.

- Is there a major psychiatric illness?
  a. Acute psychosis: Often produces major sleep disruption - treat with antipsychotics.
  b. Mania or hypomania: Very short sleep time - use antipsychotics or lithium.
  c. Major Depression: Usually there is early morning awakening but frequent awakenings during the night are also common. REM sleep begins very quickly. Treat the depression (tricyclics decrease REM sleep).

- Is there a medical problem?
  a. Chronic pain and related anxiety and depression - eg, back pain, headache, arthritis, asthma, nocturnal angina (increased pains during REM sleep), duodenal ulcer.
  b. Hyperthyroidism, epilepsy, general paresis.
  c. Is the patient simply worried about a medical problem?

- Is there substance use or abuse? Very common so always inquire.
  a. Alcohol - The most common self-prescribed hypnotic. Chronic use produces fragmented sleep.
  b. Hypnotic medication - Often prescribed by physicians for insomnia. Tolerance develops to each of them with, ironically, sleep disruption ("sleeping-pill insomnia"). Severe rebound insomnia usually occurs with withdrawal - least with the long acting benzodiazepines (eg, flurazepam). Treatment must begin with withdrawal of the medication - at the rate of one therapeutic dose/wk.
  c. Caffeine - patients often overlook. Ask.
  d. Cigarettes (nicotine) can stimulate.
  e. Amphetamines, methylphenidate, hallucinogens, aminophylline, ephedrine, and steroids all can interrupt sleep.

- Is there sleep cycle disruption? Sleepiness may become out of phase if there is "jet lag" or night shift work. Usually self-limited.

- Is there Nocturnal Myoclonus? Restless sleep with frequent awakenings secondary to muscle contractions (jerks) in the legs. Ask the bed partner. However, recent evidence suggests that nocturnal myoclonus plays little role in producing insomnia (Kales et al, 1982). There is no assured treatment but consider a trial of a small dose of clonazepam (0.5-2 mg) at bedtime.

- Is it caused by the <u>Restless Legs Syndrome</u>? Legs feel "uncomfortable" - only relieved by moving.

- Is there <u>Sleep Apnea</u> or <u>Narcolepsy</u> (see below)?

- Are there frequent <u>nightmares</u>, <u>night terrors</u> (pavor nocturnus), or <u>sleepwalking</u> (<u>somnambulism</u>)?
  a. Nightmares (REM sleep) can be chronic and disruptive - psychotherapy <u>may</u> help.
  b. Night terrors (stage 4 sleep) occur early in the night in children, are terrifying to observers, but are not remembered by the patient. They usually disappear with adulthood. Some respond to low doses of minor tranquilizers (eg, diazepam).
  c. Somnambulism (stage 4 sleep) can persist into adulthood. The patient's behavior appears strange to an observer - there is marked clouding of consciousness. Protect the patient from his actions. Diazepam, 15 mg, HS, or imipramine 50 mg, HS may help.

GENERAL TREATMENT OF INSOMNIA

1. Rule out, or treat, specific syndromes.
2. Maintain a regular bedtime. Keep room dark and quiet. Develop a "sleeping ritual." Arise promptly in the morning.
3. Regular exercise during the day helps. Avoid vigorous mental activities late in the evening. Try a bedtime snack but <u>don't</u> drink alcohol after supper.
4. Provide support and reassurance. Psychotherapy may be essential.
5. Try relaxation techniques: Progressive relaxation, biofeedback, self-hypnosis, meditation, etc.
6. Use sedative-hypnotics for a limited time only. Most hypnotic medications (exception is flurazepam) become ineffective within two weeks if used nightly. Try initially for one week in an effort to establish a successful sleep pattern (eg, flurazepam 15-30 mg, PO, HS but be aware that flurazepam can produce a gradual worsening of psychomotor performance). If used longer than a week, introduce drug holidays and don't exceed recommended dosage. There is growing evidence that naturally occurring L-tryptophan (a serotonin precursor) may relieve insomnia.

HYPERSOMNIA

1. Hypersomnia is associated more commonly with purely
   psychological causes; depression (particularly in
   younger patients), anxiety, and withdrawal. It is a
   means of escape from stress. These patients usually
   sleep excessively at night rather than during the day.

2. Does the patient have NARCOLEPSY? Narcolepsy is a
   lifelong disorder which usually begins at puberty, is
   more common in males, probably has a genetic component,
   occurs with a frequency of about 1/2000, and is
   characterized by the narcoleptic tetrad:

   a. Daytime sleep attacks - The patient falls abruptly
      asleep (REM activity on EEG) during the day, in
      spite of efforts to stay awake. He usually sleeps
      for several minutes and wakes refreshed but may have
      from several to more than 100 episodes during a day.
      The attacks are likely to occur while he is active
      and engaged and can be embarrassing or dangerous
      (during a speech, driving a car).
   b. Cataplexy - A sudden loss of muscle tone which may
      result in a fall to the ground or just a feeling of
      weakness. It usually is precipitated by a strong
      emotion (eg, anger, laughter) and can last from
      seconds to many minutes. The patient is conscious
      throughout.
   c. Hypnagogic hallucinations - Dreamlike and often
      frightening auditory and/or visual hallucinations
      which occur as the patient falls asleep or as he
      awakens (hypnopompic).
   d. Sleep paralysis - A flaccid, generalized paralysis
      lasting for several seconds in a fully conscious
      patient, either while waking or falling asleep, and
      accompanied by a strong sense of fear. It resolves
      spontaneously or when the patient is touched or his
      name is called.

Some patients suffer only sleep attacks, many also have
cataplexy (more than two-thirds), and less than 50% also
display hallucinations or sleep paralysis. 10-20% of
patients have the complete tetrad. Most patients with
narcolepsy also have disturbed nighttime sleep with
frequent awakenings and nightmares.

TREATMENT:
   1. Train the patient to avoid dangerous occupations and
      precipitating stimuli. Planned daytime naps can help.
   2. Sleep Attacks - methylphenidate (Ritalin), 5-10 mg,
      PO, TID. Insist on occasional drug holidays. This

treatment is unsatisfactory, but psychopharmacological advances are on the horizon.
3. Narcolepsy with cataplexy - add imipramine, 10-25 mg, PO, TID (suppresses REM sleep).
4. Consider sedation for insomnia (ie, benzodiazepines).

3. Does the patient have SLEEP APNEA? This serious abnormality of nighttime respiratory function can cause longstanding daytime sleepiness, particularly during quiet times (unlike narcolepsy), but is not a likely cause of insomnia (Kales et al, 1982). It occurs in three types: (1) a few patients briefly cease nighttime breathing efforts (Central Sleep Apnea), (2) the majority struggle to draw air through nose and mouth passageways which have markedly increased sleep-induced resistance (Obstructive Sleep Apnea), and (3) some suffer both phenomena (Mixed S.A.). There may be from 30 to several hundred episodes each night lasting from 10 seconds to more than two minutes. Males are affected 20:1. The patients may experience a variety of symptoms including frequent awakenings, impaired libido, loud snoring, sleepwalking, hypertension, headaches, depression, and intellectual and personality changes. Only a few cases will demonstrate anatomical abnormalities of upper airway structures. In serious chronic cases pulmonary hypertension, right heart failure, and/or cardiac arrhythmias may occur.

No treatment has been clearly effective for Central Sleep Apnea. A permanent tracheostomy may be dramatically successful in Obstructive Sleep Apnea, but try weight loss and medication (theophylline, pemoline, thioridazine) first. Hypnotics can further compromise nighttime breathing - don't use them.

4. Rule out current use of sedative drugs or rebound in chronic amphetamine users.

5. Rule out medical conditions: eg, myxedema, hypercapnia, any brain tumor but particularly those involving the mesencephalon and walls of the 3rd ventricle, seizures, cerebrovascular disease, hypoglycemia. Severe hypersomnia with marked post-awakening confusion occurs with both the Pickwickian syndrome (obesity and respiratory insufficiency) and the Kleine-Levin syndrome (attacks of hyperphagia, hypersomnia, and hypersexuality).

REFERENCES

1. Aaronson ST, Rashed S, Biber MP, Hobson JA: Brain state and body position. Arch Gen Psychiat 39:330, 1982.
2. Brownell LG, West P, Sweatman P, Acres JC, Kryger MH: Protriptyline in obstructive sleep apnea. NEJM 307:1037, 1982.
3. Coleman RM, et al: Sleep-wake disorders based on a polysomnographic diagnosis. JAMA 247:997, 1982.
4. Guilleminault C, Dement WC: Sleep Apnea Syndromes. New York, Alan Liss, 1978.
5. Kales A, Bixler EO, Soldatos CR, Vela-Bueno A, Caldwell AB, Cadieux RJ: Role of sleep apnea and nocturnal myoclonus. Psychosomatics 23:589, 1982.
6. Kreis P, Kripke DF, Ancoli-Israel S: Sleep apnea: a prospective study. West J Med 139:171, 1983.
7. Orr WC, Altshuler KZ, Stahl ML: Managing Sleep Complaints. Chicago, Year Book Med Pub, 1982.
8. Piccione P, Tallarigo R, Zorick R, Wittig R, Roth R: Personality differences between insomniac and non-insomniac psychiatry outpatients. J Clin Psychiat 42:261, 1981.
9. Sleeping Pills, Insomnia, and Medical Practice. National Academy of Sciences, Institute of Medicine, Division of Mental Health and Behavioral Medicine, 1979.
10. Soldatos CR, Kales A, Kales JD: Management of insomnia. Ann Rev Med 30:301, 1979.
11. Williams RL, Karacan I: Sleep Disorders: Diagnosis and Treatment. New York, John Wiley & Sons, 1978.

Chapter 21

Mental Retardation

There are 6,000,000 mentally retarded persons in the USA of which 80-85% are only mildly retarded. Retardation is a clinical phenomenon reflecting general intellectual functioning (IQ), social and occupational adaptation, maturation and age, and the environmental and cultural setting. Adults with intellectual impairment which developed before age 18 are considered retarded. Impairment occuring after 18 is dementia.

APA CLASSIFICATION

MILD MENTAL RETARDATION (DSM-III p 39, 317.0) - IQ 50-70. Usually recognized when they enter school - requires special education. The majority become self-supporting. The prevalence of this diagnosis decreases markedly with adulthood.

MODERATE MENTAL RETARDATION (DSM-III p 39, 318.0) - IQ 35-49. They are trainable, can learn simple work skills, and can be partly self-supporting in sheltered settings.

SEVERE MENTAL RETARDATION (DSM-III p 39, 318.1) - IQ 20-34. 7% of all retarded. They are capable of simple speech but require institutional or other intensely supportive care.

PROFOUND MENTAL RETARDATION (DSM-III p 39, 318.2) - IQ below 20. 1% of all retarded. They are totally dependent upon others for survival.

A presumably retarded patient who is untestable is considered to have UNSPECIFIED MENTAL RETARDATION (DSM-III p 40, 319.0).

CAUSES

Distinct causes (usually biological) are identified for only 25% of patients and those occur predominantly in the moderately to profoundly retarded patients. The

rest appear to be due to environmental factors with an
uncertain polygenetic contribution in some cases.
Moderate to profound retardation is distributed uniformly
across social classes while mild retardation is almost
specific to the lower classes.

Major biological causes include:

Chromosomal abnormalities - numerous types including
  Down's Syndrome (mongolism, trisomy 21), Cri Du Chat
  Syndrome, Klinefelter's Syndrome (XXY), Turner's
  Syndrome (XO/XX).
Dominant genetic inheritance - Neurofibromatosis
  (Von Recklinghausen's Disease), Huntington's
  Chorea, Marfan's Syndrome, Sturge-Weber Syndrome,
  Tuberous Sclerosis.
Metabolic disorders - Phenylketonuria (PKU), Hartnup
  Disease, fructose intolerance, galactosemia,
  Wilson's Disease, a variety of lipid disorders,
  hypothyroidism, hypoglycemia.
Prenatal disorders - maternal rubella (particularly in
  the 1st trimester), syphilis, toxoplasmosis, or
  diabetes; maternal alcohol abuse (Fetal Alcohol
  Syndrome) and use of some drugs (eg, thalidomide);
  toxemia of pregnancy; erythroblastosis fetalis;
  maternal malnutrition.
Birth trauma - difficult delivery with physical trauma
  and/or anoxia, prematurity.
Brain trauma - tumors, infection (particularly
  encephalitis, neonatal meningitis), accidents,
  poisons (eg, lead, mercury), hydrocephalus, numerous
  types of cranial abnormalities.

Social causes include substandard education, environmental
  deprivation, childhood abuse and neglect,
  restricted activity.

Rule out Specific and Pervasive Developmental
Disorders, dementia, and Residual Schizophrenia. Rule
out BORDERLINE INTELLECTUAL FUNCTION (DSM-III p 332,
V62.89). Look for associated psychiatric or neurological
syndromes.

TREATMENT AND PROGNOSIS

Most mildly retarded individuals demonstrate
significantly improved functioning with education and a
supportive environment. They are at risk for adjustment
reaction, depression, psychotic reactions, and behavioral
disturbances 2° to a negative self-image. Treat the
patient with supportive, reality oriented psychotherapy.
Determine the patient's coping style and temperamental

strengths and encourage them but don't demand too much. Simple behavior modification techniques may be very effective and should be part of any treatment program. Low doses of minor or major tranquilizers may help behavior problems (eg, aggressiveness) - don't overuse (It's easy to do). Lithium may moderate aggression in some cases.

Severely retarded persons may require some form of institutionalization, yet training in sheltered settings should be considered.

If the patient lives with his family - treat the family. Parents and siblings frequently display anger, rejection, overprotection and overcontrol, denial, and/or guilt - all of which should be recognized and dealt with by the physician. Provide genetic counseling. Coordinate with outside agencies and specialists, when available.

The majority of mildly retarded adults are indistinguishable from the general population, thus prognosis is good for a productive, self-sufficient life. Mild mental retardation is not incurable.

REFERENCES

1. Bowlby J: Maternal Care and Mental Health. Geneva, World Health Organization, 1951.
2. Carter CH: Medical Aspects of Mental Retardation, ed 2. Springfield, Charles C Thomas Pub, 1978.
3. Eaton LF, Menolascino FJ: Psychiatric disorders in the mentally retarded: types, problems, and challenges. Am J Psychiat 139:1297, 1982.
4. Schwartz M, Duara R, Haxby J, Grady C, White BJ, Kessler RM, Kay AD, Cutler NR, Rapoport SI: Down's syndrome in adults: brain metabolism. Science 221:781, 1983.
5. Tu J: A survey of psychotropic medication in mental retardation facilities. J Clin Psychiat 40:125, 1979.

Chapter 22

The Psychotherapies

There are dozens of different psychotherapies address-
ing innumerable different patient problems. With the
possible exception of a few specific behavioral methods
applied to several very limited and discrete problems,
rigorous proof of psychotherapy's effectiveness is not
available. However, there is much non-rigorous but very
compelling experience which indicates that various
psychotherapies can help many patients. Unfortunately,
specific indications for specific therapies generally are
not currently available (Beutler, 1979). Some experts
argue that many supposedly different psychotherapeutic
methods are actually quite similar in practice (eg, Brunink
and Schroeder, 1979). Others suggest that trained
therapists utilizing specific techniques may be less
important for the patient's improvement than the
therapist's personal characteristics of accurate empathy,
non-possessive warmth, and genuineness (Strupp and Hadley,
1979).

Although there remain more questions than answers
about the utility of and indications for psychotherapy and
it is a field which has yet to reach a high level of
scientific objectivity, it is clear that some patients
benefit from such care and that an essential ingredient to
that care is a good patient-therapist relationship built on
trust and genuine interest. Psychotherapy is an art and a
good therapist does make a difference.

INDIVIDUAL THERAPY

Individual treatment is the most common form of
psychotherapy and comes in almost endless variations. The
two most common types available in the USA are:

SUPPORTIVE THERAPY:

This is the most typical form of individual therapy provided to inpatients and outpatients. Therapists skilled in this method include psychiatrists, clinical psychologists, and social workers. The goal is to evaluate the patient's current life situation and his strengths and weaknesses and then to help him make whatever realistic changes will allow him to be more functional. Patients usually are seen weekly (or more often) for several weeks or months (although some patients are followed infrequently for years). Also included is brief (1-3 session) crisis intervention.

The therapist deals with the patient's symptoms but works very little with the patient's unconscious processes and does not attempt major personality change. Psychological defenses are reinforced - techniques used include reassurance, suggestion, ventilation, abreaction, and environmental manipulation. The therapist must be active, interested, empathic, and warm - listen to the patient, understand his concerns, and help him find direction. Medication may be used.

Patients who are failing to cope successfully with present stress are good candidates, whether or not they have underlying psychiatric problems. Patients with serious psychiatric illnesses (eg, schizophrenia, major affective disorder) often benefit by concurrent use of biological methods and supportive psychotherapy.

PSYCHOANALYTIC PSYCHOTHERAPY:

Psychoanalysis is the classic, long-term insight oriented therapy. The goal is to make major personality changes by identifying and modifying ("working through") unconscious conflicts by means of free association, analysis of transference and resistance, and dream interpretation. An "analysis" typically takes several hundred hours. "Neurotics" and those with personality disorders are the preferred patients.

Psychoanalytic psychotherapy (as distinguished from psychoanalysis) is similar to supportive therapy in that the goal is removal of symptoms yet is similar to psychoanalysis in requiring a dynamic understanding of the patient's unconscious conflicts (insight) and in utilizing analysis of the transference and dream interpretation. It is briefer than psychoanalysis and more frequently done.

BEHAVIOR THERAPY

Over the last twenty years behavior therapy has become one of the major therapeutic modalities available to psychiatrists. It is based on learning theory which postulates that problem behaviors (ie, almost any of the manifestations of psychiatric conditions) are involuntarily acquired due to inappropriate learning. Therapy concentrates on changing behavior (behavior modification) rather than changing unconscious or conscious thought patterns and to that end it is very directive (ie, patient receives much instruction and direction). Specific techniques to facilitate those changes include the following.

Operant conditioning - These therapeutic techniques are based on careful evaluation and modification of the antecedents and consequences of a patient's behavior. Desired behavior is encouraged by positive reinforcement and discouraged by negative reinforcement. These new ways of responding to the patient can be taught to the people who live with the patient or, for inpatients, may take the form of a token economy.

Aversion therapy - A patient is given an unpleasant, aversive stimulus (eg, electric shock, loud sound) when his behavior is undesirable. Some of these procedures have been legally discouraged. An alternate technique, covert sensitization, is less objectionable since it uses the patient's unpleasant thoughts as the aversive stimulus.

Implosive therapy - The patient with a situation-caused anxiety is directly exposed for a length of time to that situation (flooding) or exposed in imagination (implosion). The anxiety is frequently relieved.

Systematic desensitization - The anxious or phobic patient is exposed to a gradual hierarchy of frightening situations or objects, beginning with the least worrisome. He gradually learns to handle the more frightening ones. If this is paired with relaxation (ie, an antagonistic response pattern - relaxation is incompatible with anxiety), the technique is reciprocal inhibition.

Common to these methods (and numerous others) is rigorous data collection. Behavior therapy relies on careful measurement of behavior. A technique is considered useful only if it is successful and its success is determined by whether it eliminates measurable undesirable behavior or increases desirable behavior.

Although behavior modification has been successful in treating some kinds of conditions (eg, phobias, sexual deviance, regressed behavior), it has been criticized for not considering thought processes. This has led to broader conceptualizations including Cognitive Behavior Modification (eg, Rehm, 1981) and Multimodal Behavior Therapy (Lazarus, 1981).

GROUP THERAPY
_____

Group therapy comes in many different forms - most of them derived from different types of individual therapy.

Interpersonal exploration groups - The goal is to develop self-awareness of interpersonal styles through corrective feedback from other group members. Patient is accepted and supported, thus promoting self-esteem. It is the most common type of group therapy.

Guidance-inspirational groups - Highly structured, cohesive, supportive groups which minimize the importance of insight and maximize the value of ventilation and camaraderie. Groups may be large - eg, Alcoholics Anonymous (AA), Synanon. Members often are chosen because they "have the same problem."

Psychoanalytically oriented therapy - A loosely structured group technique in which the therapist makes interpretations about a patient's unconscious conflicts and processes from observed group interactions.

Numerous other types of group therapies include behavioral therapy, Gestalt, encounter, psychodrama, transactional analysis (TA), marathon, EST, etc.

Groups may run for several weeks or several years, usually weekly. They usually have 5-12 members (depending on type). Therapists from many different disciplines conduct groups - many groups run with co-therapists.

Some groups have patients with only one diagnosis (eg, schizophrenia, alcoholism) while others are mixed. It is not clear which patients will benefit (or will be harmed) by group therapy but most patients can be treated safely in groups. Most of the success of a group appears to depend more on the experience, sensitivity, warmth, and charisma of the leader than on the group's theoretical orientation.

A group experience which is too intense or confrontive can produce anxiety, depressive, or psychotic reactions in susceptible patients. Acutely psychotic patients should not be included. Paranoid individuals make poor group members.

FAMILY THERAPY:

Family therapy can be conceptualized as a variant of group therapy. There are numerous types of family therapy but no "one right way." Although a family often enters therapy because one of the family members is "having problems," it is the implicit or explicit assumption of many family therapists that the system is sick, not the patient. The expectation is that improvement in unhealthy interpersonal interactions and communications will result in improvement of the identified patient.

Most (but not all) family therapists recognize that some patients bring problems to family therapy which are not due to family malfunctioning but most therapists argue that those problems are frequently worsened by any untreated malfunctioning.

MARITAL THERAPY:

Therapy of a married couple is often called for if that is the relationship at risk. It is particularly common if there is a psychosexual problem present. Theoretical orientations and treatment techniques are diverse - none has been clearly shown to be superior. There are no clear guidelines for choosing couples likely to improve with marital therapy. Therapists may come from one of several professional disciplines (eg, psychiatry, psychology, social work, marriage and family counseling).

MILIEU THERAPY:

Milieu therapy usually takes place in an inpatient "therapeutic community." Often the entire community is geared towards support for the patient and towards helping him develop more adaptive coping skills. In a sense, all the staff members are therapists and all the patients are likewise concerned with facilitating each other's well-being. It is a useful adjunct to other forms of therapy (eg, pharmacotherapy).

REFERENCES

1. Ackerman NW: The Psychodynamics of Family Life, New York, Basic Books, 1958.
2. Beutler LE: Toward specific psychological therapies for specific conditions. J Consult and Clin Psychology 47:882, 1979.
3. Brunink SA, Schroeder HE: Verbal therapeutic behavior of expert psychoanalytically oriented, gestalt, and

behavior therapists. J Consult and Clin Psychology 47:567, 1979.

4. Childress AR, Burns DD: The basics of cognitive therapy. Psychosomatics 22:1017, 1981.

5. Clark DH: The therapeutic community. Brit J Psychiat 131:553, 1977.

6. Clarkin JF, Frances A: Selection criteria for the brief psychotherapies. Am J Psychotherapy 36:166, 1982.

7. DeWitt KN, Kaltreider NB, Weiss DS, Horowitz MJ: Judging change in psychotherapy. Arch Gen Psychiat 40:1121, 1983.

8. Frank JD: Persuasion and Healing. Baltimore, The Johns Hopkins Univ Pr, 1973.

9. Garber J, Seligman MEP: Human Helplessness. New York, Academic Pr, 1980.

10. Garfield SL, Bergin AE: Handbook of Psychotherapy and Behavior Change. New York, J Wiley and Sons, 1978.

11. Kandel ER: Psychotherapy and the single synapse. NEJM 301:1028, 1979.

12. Lazarus AA: The Practice of Multimodal Therapy. New York, McGraw-Hill, 1981.

13. Malan DH: Individual Psychotherapy and the Science of Psychodynamics. London, Butterworths, 1979.

14. Marmor J: Recent trends in psychotherapy. Am J Psychiat 137:409, 1980.

15. Rehm LP: Behavior Therapy for Depression. New York, Academic Pr, 1981.

16. Rose SD: Group Therapy: A Behavioral Approach. Englewood Cliffs, Prentice-Hall Inc, 1977.

17. Satir V: Conjoint Family Therapy. Palo Alto, Science and Behavior Books Inc, 1967.

18. Smith ML, Glass GV, Miller TI: The Benefits of Psychotherapy. Baltimore, The Johns Hopkins Univ Pr, 1980.

19. Stravynski A, Marks I, Yule W: Social skills problems in neurotic outpatients. Arch Gen Psychiat 39:1378, 1982.

20. Strupp HH, Hadley SW: Specific vs nonspecific factors in psychotherapy. Arch Gen Psychiat 36:1125, 1979.

21. Wolberg LR: The Technique of Psychotherapy, 3rd ed. New York, Grune and Stratton, 1977.

22. Yalom ID: The Theory and Practice of Group Psychotherapy. New York, Basic Books, 1975.

Chapter 23

Biological Therapy

ANTIPSYCHOTICS (NEUROLEPTICS)

These are the "major tranquilizers" which revolution-
ized psychiatry by providing an effective treatment for
large numbers of psychotic patients. Their antipsychotic
effect is <u>not</u> due to sedation but to a specific action on
the thought and mood disorder.

DRUGS AVAILABLE:

There are many different antipsychotics available
which are divided among five chemical classes. Common
examples of each class are listed below along with
relative dosages (with reference to chlorpromazine).

TRICYCLICS

PHENOTHIAZINES	Equivalent doses (mg)
Dimethylamino-alkyl Derivatives	
chlorpromazine (Thorazine)	100
triflupromazine (Vesprin)	30
Piperidine-alkyl Derivatives	
thioridazine (Mellaril)	100
mesoridazine (Serentil)	50
Piperazine-alkyl Derivatives	
fluphenazine (Prolixin, Permitil)	1-1.5
fluphenazine decanoate (long-acting)	
trifluoperazine (Stelazine)	8
perphenazine (Trilafon)	10
THIOXANTHENES	
chlorprothixene (Taractan)	100
thiothixene (Navane)	8

DIBENZOXAZEPINES
        loxapine succinate (Loxitane)   15

NON-TRICYCLICS

DIHYDROINDOLONES
        molindone (Moban)   20

BUTYROPHENONES
        haloperidol (Haldol)   1-2

INDICATIONS FOR USE:
        Recommended for:

1. Acute schizophrenia and other acute psychoses (eg, amphetamine psychosis, psychoses with OBS). Should be used in conjunction with lithium in the acute manic attacks of bipolar disorder.
2. Chronic schizophrenia.
3. Major depression with significant psychotic features – used in conjunction with an anti-depressant.
4. Gilles de la Tourette Syndrome – haloperidol is the drug of choice.

Other uses:

- Antipsychotics can be of temporary use in several conditions – eg, acute agitation of a non-psychotic nature, antiemesis, etc.

MECHANISMS OF ACTION:

        The dopamine hypothesis postulates that schizophrenia is secondary to increased central dopamine activity. Antipsychotic drugs are felt to act by a postsynaptic blocking of DA receptors, thus returning a CNS DA balance. The three major CNS dopamine pathways with their associated activities are:

        Nigrostriatal – extrapyramidal actions
        Tuberoinfundibular – endocrine actions (increased
            prolactin)
        Mesolimbic – antipsychotic actions

The different side effect patterns of the various antipsychotic drugs are felt to be due to their different locations of primary activity. However, antipsychotics also block central noradrenergic (NE) receptors, thus we can't yet determine whether DA- or NE-blockage (or another mechanism entirely) is responsible for the antipsychotic effect.

PHARMACOKINETICS:

Chlorpromazine is variably absorbed from the intestine and is probably partly degraded in the mucosal wall. It is approximately 95% protein bound. Much higher blood levels are attained following IM or IV than PO administration. The half-life is 1-2$^+$ days but variable, with the majority of the drug stored in body fat. There is marked interindividual differences in blood levels (reasons are not certain).

All tricyclic antipsychotic drug metabolism is very complex (eg, chlorpromazine is degraded by sulfoxidation, hydroxylation, deamination, demethylation, etc, to form well over 100 metabolites). Some of the metabolites are active, some inactive - not completely worked out (eg, antipsychotic chlorpromazine is excreted in urine as a glucuronide). In part because of this complexity, measured plasma levels are not currently clinically useful. A better measure may be RBC drug level (still a research procedure). In contrast, non-tricyclic antipsychotics (eg, Haldol, Moban) have a simple metabolism.

SIDE EFFECTS:

Side effects are common and are almost unavoidable at higher drug dosages. The particular pattern of side effects is in part determined by the chemical class of any given antipsychotic.

Drug	Sedation	Extrapyramidal	Hypotension
Phenothiazines			
Aliphatic	3+	2+	3+
Piperidine	2+	1+	2+
Piperazine	1+	3+	1+
Dibenzoxazepines	2+	3+	2+
Butyrophenones	2+	3+	1+
Dihydroindolones	1+	2+	1+

These side effects also have marked interindividual variability. The most common side effects of these medications include sedation, extrapyramidal and anticholinergic symptoms, hypotension, weight gain, and reduced libido but there are a large number of other side effects which may be encountered.

- Sedation: Common; use a QD schedule, if possible.

- Anticholinergic symptoms:
     Dry mouth - Common. May lead to moniliasis,
          parotitis, and increase in cavities. Consider

treatment with oral water and ice, sugarless
gum; also neostigmine 7.5-15 mg PO, pilocarpine
2.5 mg PO QID, or bethanechol 75 mg daily.
Constipation - Treat with stool softeners.
Blurred vision - Near vision. Treat with physostigmine drops, 0.25% solution, 1 drop Q6H, if
a major problem.
Urinary hesitancy and retention - Consider using
Urecholine 10-25 mg PO TID.
Exacerbation of glaucoma
Central anticholinergic syndrome - Occurs particularly
in those patients simultaneously taking several
drugs with anticholinergic properties (eg,
an OD or a patient taking an antipsychotic, an
antidepressant, and an antiparkinsonian). The
syndrome can vary from mild anxiety and vaso-
dilatation to a toxic delirium or even coma. It
is much more common in the elderly. Symptoms
and signs to be looked for include:

Anxiety, restlessness, agitation - grading
into confusion, incoherence, disorientation,
memory impairment, visual and auditory
hallucinations - grading into seizures,
stupor, and coma.
Warm and dry skin, flushed face, dry mouth,
hyperpyrexia.
Blurred vision, dilated pupils.
Absent bowel sounds.

Treat an acute delirium with withdrawal of the
causative agent, close medical supervision
(eg, cardiac monitor), and physostigmine 1-2 mg
IM or slowly IV (eg, 1 mg/min). Repeat in 15 - 30
min and then every 1-2 hours, if needed. Avoid
physostigmine in patients with bowel or bladder
obstruction, peptic ulcer, asthma, glaucoma,
heart disease, diabetes, or hypothyroidism.
Watch for cholinergic overdosage (salivation,
sweating, etc) and treat with atropine (0.5 mg
for each mg of physostigmine).

- Extrapyramidal symptoms: These reactions are common,
get worse with stress, disappear during sleep, and
wax and wane over time.

Acute dystonic reaction - An involuntary, sustained
contraction of a skeletal muscle which usually
appears suddenly (over 5-60 minutes). The jaw
muscles are most frequently involved (ie,
"lock-jaw") but other muscle systems may also

be disturbed (eg, torticollis, carpopedal spasm, oculogyric crisis, even opisthotonos). Usually occurs during the first two days of treatment (in 2-10% of patients - more common in younger patients.

Parkinson-like syndrome - These reactions occur individually or together, usually during weeks 1-4 of treatment. They are more common in older patients.

Tremor - An irregular tremor of the upper extremities, tongue, and jaw. It occurs with both movement and rest and is slower than the tremors produced by TCA and lithium.

Rigidity - A cogwheel rigidity which starts with the shoulders and spreads to the upper extremities and then throughout the body.

Akinesia - A "zombie-like" effect with slowness, fatigue, micrographia, and little facial expression. It may occur alone and at anytime during the course of treatment and is easily mistaken for social withdrawal or depression.

Akathisia: Common and resistant to treatment. Patients are fidgety, constantly move their hands and feet, rock from the waist, and shift from foot to foot. Easily mistaken for anxiety or agitation.

Rabbit Syndrome: Involuntary chewing movements.

Tardive dyskinesia: Slow choreiform or tic-like movements, usually of the tongue and facial muscles, but occasionally of the upper extremities or the whole body. Risk is increased in the aged, those with OBS, females, high doses of medication, simultaneous use of several antipsychotics, and possibly long duration of treatment. Develops over months or years of antipsychotic use and the more severe cases are often irreversible (perhaps as high as 25% of affected patients). Symptoms disappear with an increased dosage of antipsychotic - don't "misread" the movements as a worsening psychosis, raise the dose of medication, remove the symptom, and thus begin a vicious cycle. "Drug holidays" don't seem to prevent, and may even worsen, the development of TD (Branchey and Branchey, 1984). There is no acceptable treatment. Try to discontinue the antipsychotic, if possible.

TREATMENT OF EXTRAPYRAMIDAL SYMPTOMS

Treat with the anticholinergic <u>antiparkinsonism drugs</u>
(see review by McEvoy, 1983):

Drug	Typical Dosage
benztropine (Cogentin)	1-4 mg, QD-BID, PO
biperiden (Akineton)	1-2 mg, TID-QID, PO
procyclidine (Kemadrin)	2-5 mg, TID-QID, PO
trihexyphenidyl (Artane, Tremin)	2-5 mg, TID-QID, PO
diphenhydramine (Benadryl)	25-50 mg, TID-QID, PO

Begin at a lower dosage and raise over several days.
Use for several weeks, then discontinue if possible. Try
not to use for more than 2-3 months (although they may be
necessary long-term in a few patients - see Van Putten,
1983). Some studies support the use of antiparkinsonism
drugs prophylactically (begun when antipsychotics are
started), particularly in patients likely to be resistant
(Keepers et al, 1983). Treat acute dystonic reactions
immediately (IM or IV) with (eg) Cogentin 1 mg, Benadryl
25-50 mg, or Valium 5-10 mg - then begin regular oral dose
for several weeks.

- Alpha-adrenergic blocking symptoms: Orthostatic
    hypotension, inhibition of ejaculation (particularly
    thioridazine).

- Cholestatic jaundice: Probably a sensitivity reaction.
    Fever and eosinophilia, usually during the first two
    months of treatment (in 1% of patients taking
    chlorpromazine). Little cross-sensitivity with other
    antipsychotics.

- Agranulocytosis: Usually in elderly females during the
    first four months of treatment but can occur anytime.
    Train patients to report persistent sore throats,
    infections, or fever. Rare.

- Neuroleptic Malignant Syndrome (NMS): Infrequent;
    usually but not exclusively following high dose IM
    treatment. Symptoms develop rapidly and include
    marked muscular rigidity, clouded consciousness,
    hyperthermia, hypertension, diaphoresis, and
    tachycardia. Very dangerous - stop medication
    immediately and provide medical support. Patient may
    recover over 5-15 days.

- Hypothermia; hyperthermia: Watch out for hot seclusion
    rooms.

- Weight gain, obesity.

- Pigmentary changes in skin: Particularly with chlorpromazine. A tan, gray, or blue color.

- Retinitis Pigmentosa - Possible blindness. Occurs with
  dosages of thioridazine greater than 800 mg/day.

- Photosensitivity: Bad sunburns with Thorazine.

- Grand mal seizures: Particularly with rapid increases in
  dose.

- Non-specific skin rashes: In 5%.

- Reduced libido in males and females.

- Increased prolactin levels: Produces galactorrhea,
  amenorrhea, and lactation.

- EKG changes: Particularly with thioridazine - T-wave
  inversions, occasionally arrhythmias.

- Appears safe during pregnancy: no known congenital
  abnormalities. Slight hypertonicity among newborns,
  but little effect on nursing infant.

  Suicide is difficult but possible with the antipsychotics - requires very large doses.

DRUG INTERACTIONS:

  Antacids - May inhibit absorption of oral antipsychotics.
  Tricyclic antidepressants - May inhibit antipsychotic
    metabolism and raise plasma levels, and vice versa.

TREATMENT PRINCIPLES:

- Drug choice:

    The primary reason to choose one drug over another
  is the side effect spectrum - they are all equally
  capable of controlling psychosis when given in
  appropriate doses. If a patient or a similarly
  affected family member has responded well to one
  medication, try it. If a patient has a seizure
  disorder, use a high potency drug (eg, fluphenazine,
  haloperidol).

- Treatment of acute psychosis:

     Sedating antipsychotics which can be given IM
     usually provide the best control initially (eg,
     Haldol, Thorazine), although they have no long-term
     advantages. Give orally if the patient is cooperative
     - IM if he is not.

     1. If possible, give a small test dose (eg, Haldol 5
        mg) and wait one hour to see if it is tolerated.
     2. Then begin Haldol 10-20 mg/day, Thorazine 300-400
        mg/day, or the equivalent. Use TID or QID
        schedule initially, then switch to BID or QD
        after 1-2 weeks. A QD schedule is usually well
        tolerated and helps insomnia. Increase the
        equivalent of 100-200 mg of Thorazine every 3-4
        days until the patient has improved or side
        effects become limiting. Maximum dosages needed
        are highly variable (may be as high as 1500-2000
        mg of chlorpromazine, or more). If side effects
        become a problem, begin antiparkinsonism drugs
        and/or reduce the dosage and increase more slowly.
     3. If the patient is wild and needs immediate control,
        consider "rapid tranquilization" with
        antipsychotics - eg:

          Haldol 5 mg IM every hour until calm (maximum
             50 mg in 12 hrs), or

          Thorazine 50 mg PO, then 100 mg/hr, max 6-8 hr

          Monitor carefully for hypotension or oversedation.
          Once the patient is under control, switch to the
          preceding daily schedule.

- Disease control is cognitive as well as behavioral - the
  goal is not just to "quiet" the patient. Increasing
  socialization is an early sign of a drug response.
  Agitated, disruptive behavior usually improves in the
  first several days with the thought disorder dis-
  appearing over weeks or months. Although antipsychotics improve "active" psychotic symptoms (eg, hallucinations, delusions, bizarre behavior), they usually
  don't change the patient's basic personality or the
  "passive" symptoms (eg, flat affect, social impairment).
  Patients who are "acutely crazy" are most likely to
  respond well, as are those with good premorbid
  functioning who are having their first psychotic
  episode.

- If a patient does not respond, switch to another drug of

a different class. However, the unimproved patient
needs at least one 2-3 week trial at a high dose of an
antipsychotic before you conclude that he doesn't
respond to medication. There is rarely a reason to
use two different antipsychotics simultaneously. The
most common cause for lack of response is underdosage
(and noncompliance), but always be wary that the
patient may have an organic psychosis.

- Once improvement has occurred, maintain drug levels over
  1-2 months and then consider reducing to maintenance
  levels. If this is the first episode of an acute
  psychosis in a previously well-functioning patient,
  consider discontinuing the medication over another 1-2
  months. If this episode is one of many, place on
  maintenance.

- Antipsychotic maintenance therapy:

    Decrease dosage slowly (over weeks - months) to
    one third or one quarter of the acute dose. Depending
    on past history, try discontinuing after 6-12 months
    although there is recent evidence that some patients
    may need meds for many years. If a relapse develops,
    increase the dose. 80-90% of patients relapse (during
    first 24 months) without meds, 40% relapse while
    taking them. Teach the patient to recognize his own
    developing relapse so it can be caught early. Try
    occasional "drug holidays" - ie, no medication during
    occasional weeks or weekends.

- Antipsychotics are often unpleasant to take, so compliance
  is a major problem with outpatients (particularly in
  those patients who are suspicious and paranoid). Pay
  attention to and work aggressively to control side
  effects (particularly akathisia - see Van Putten et
  al, 1984). A major recent advance has been the
  development of a long-acting depot form of fluphenazine (Prolixin decanoate). A maintenance dose can be
  given by shot every several weeks (eg, Prolixin decanoate 0.5-2.5 cc IM, every 2-3 weeks), thus assuring the
  therapist that the patient is receiving his
  medication. Lowering the dose may increase the risk
  of relapse but decrease the risk of tardive dyskinesia
  (Kane et al, 1983).

- Abrupt medication withdrawal may produce symptoms (for 1-
  2 weeks) of cholinergic rebound (eg, sweating,
  abdominal cramps, diarrhea, nausea) and CNS
  stimulation (eg, tremor, restlessness, insomnia).

LITHIUM CARBONATE

DRUGS AVAILABLE:

Lithium carbonate (Li^+ - atomic # 3)

INDICATIONS FOR USE:

Recommended for:

1. Acute bipolar disorder, manic. Lithium is clearly
   the drug of choice for an acute manic attack
   (80% of patients return to normal) although, due
   to the usual 7-10 day delay in onset of clinical
   effect, a major tranquilizer may be needed
   initially as well.
2. Used with an antidepressant in acute depression in
   a bipolar patient to prevent "manic overshoot."
3. Long-term prophylaxis of mania in a bipolar patient.
   It is effective at preventing recurrences. Be
   careful of chronic renal toxicity.

Possible uses:

- Prophylaxis for bipolar disorder, depressed and for
  major depression.
- May be an effective antidepressant for some patients
  with an acute bipolar depression. It may act
  synergistically with tricyclic antidepressants.
- May assist or replace antipsychotics in treatment of
  some patients with schizophrenia or schizoaffective disorder (but lithium can make a few
  schizophrenics worse).
- May help control mood swings and explosive outbursts
  in patients with intermittent explosive disorder
  and emotionally unstable character disorder.
- Retarded patients with aggressiveness and/or self-
  mutilation.

MECHANISMS OF ACTION:

The reasons for the clinical effects are unknown
although it does increase central NE reuptake and decrease
its release.

PHARMACOKINETICS:

Lithium is quickly absorbed from the GI tract
(completely absorbed in 8 hours) and develops a peak plasma
level in 1-3 hours. It is not protein bound
or metabolized and is excreted by the kidney. The CSF

concentration is 30-60% of that in plasma and equivalent to that in RBCs. It is concentrated by bone and by thyroid (4-5 X that in plasma).

Lithium can only be used safely if blood concentrations are monitored carefully (oral dosage is not an adequate measure). To obtain consistent levels, blood is routinely drawn 12 hrs after the last dose (usually before breakfast). The lithium half-life is 18-36 hrs (fastest in youth, slowest in elderly) - a constant oral dosage requires 5-8 days to reach steady state. Once a steady state is reached, the lithium level is proportional to the daily oral dose (and determined by the renal clearance).

SIDE EFFECTS:

The number and severity of side effects increase with increasing or rapidly changing blood levels. Minor side effects (tremor, thirst, anorexia and GI distress) commonly occur at therapeutic levels (0.8-1.5 meq/l) and fatal effects (seizures, coma) may occur at only slightly higher levels (eg, as low as 2.0-2.5 meq/l but more commonly at 3-5 meq/l). Lithium has a very narrow margin of safety and is a dangerous drug in overdosage. It should be given cautiously (or not given at all) in patients who are dehydrated, have sodium depletion (kidney reabsorbs more lithium), or have major renal or cardiovascular disease. Brain damaged patients and the elderly are at risk for side effects at low blood levels.

Normal subjects administered lithium report irritability and emotional lability, anxiety, mild depression, tiredness and malaise, weakness, inability to concentrate, and slowed reaction time. Patients taking lithium often experience a "lithium-induced dysphoria" - 25-50% stop lithium AMA. Unlike other psychoactive medication, sedation is not a side effect.

Neurological:
    EEG - Usually shows increased amplitude and generalized
        slowing (in 50% of patients at therapeutic blood
        levels).
    Headaches, occasional slurred speech.
    Toxicity:
        Confusion, poor concentration, and clouding of
            consciousness; leads to delirium; leads to
            coma; leads to death.
        Cerebellar effects - dysarthria, ataxia,
            nystagmus, severe incoordination.
        Basal ganglia effects - Parkinsonian symptoms,
            choreiform movements.
        Seizures - grand mal; status epilipticus.

Neuromuscular:
>   Hand tremor (fine, fast) which does not respond to
>   anticholinergics. Occurs in 50% of the patients
>   started on lithium but the incidence decreases
>   with time (5% of long-term patients).
>   Muscular weakness - one third of patients during the
>   first week of treatment; transient.
>   Neuromuscular toxicity - hyperactive reflexes,
>   fasciculations, paralysis.

Kidney:
>   Polyuria and polydipsia - secondary to a vasopressin-
>   resistant, diabetes insipidus-like syndrome.
>   Reversible and occurs in 50% of all new patients
>   (5% of all chronics).
>   Reversible oliguric renal failure with acute lithium
>   intoxication.
>   Possible irreversible nephrotoxic effect in a few
>   chronic patients - focal interstitial cortical
>   fibrosis with tubular atrophy and sclerotic
>   glomeruli. Look for a gradually increasing blood
>   lithium in patients taking a constant oral dose.
>   There is increased serum creatinine and an
>   increased 24 hr urine volume. Poorly character-
>   ized currently, this serious effect of chronic
>   lithium administration may ultimately limit the
>   ability to use lithium prophylactically in some.

Blood:
>   Leukocytosis (10,000-14,000 WBCs - neutrophilia with
>   lymphocytopenia). Common and reversible, it is
>   persistent but periodic while the patient is
>   taking lithium.
>   Occasional increased ESR.

GI:
>   30% of patients have GI symptoms in the early weeks of
>   treatment - gastric irritation, nausea, anorexia,
>   diarrhea, bloating, abdominal pain (a switch to
>   lithium citrate may relieve symptoms).

Heart:
>   T-wave flattening or inversion (common but reversible).
>   Unusual - myocarditis, SA block, primary AV block;
>   ventricular irritability and perhaps sudden death
>   (particularly in older males with cardiac
>   pathology; more common at toxic levels).

Thyroid:
>   Lithium may produce a goiter in 10% of chronic
>   patients - a variety of types (eg, euthyroid

goiter, goiter with hypothyroidism). There may
also be hypothyroidism without a goiter. Consult
an endocrinologist if a goiter develops.

Other:
Lithium accumulates in bone - no known harmful effects.
Occasional maculopapular rash, acne - also rare
alopecia, ulceration, and exacerbation of
psoriasis.
Weight gain in 10% of patients.
Both decreased and increased glucose tolerance can
occur as well as an elevated blood sugar.
Occasional benign, reversible exophthalmos.
Hyperparathyroidism - increased serum calcium and
parathyroid hormone, usually without other
symptoms.

Most of the side effects disappear with chronic lithium
administration. Persistent side effects include tremor,
polyuria, leukocytosis, goiter, and elevated blood sugar.

In Pregnancy:

1. Lithium crosses the placenta freely and perhaps
produces cardiac malformations - thus, pregnant
women should not take lithium unless they absolutely
must. Such infants are also at risk for nephrogenic
diabetes insipidus, hypoglycemia, and euthyroid
goiter.
2. Lithium in milk is 30-100% of the maternal blood level
- thus, these mothers should not breast feed.
3. Lithium clearance increases 50-100% early in pregnancy
and returns to normal at delivery; so a dosage which
had been raised during pregnancy must be immediately
reduced or the mother will become toxic.

DRUG INTERACTIONS:

Diuretics - Thiazides decrease lithium clearance and
increase blood levels. Furosemide, ethacrynic acid,
spironolactone, and triamterene may also. Mannitol,
urea, and acetazolamide decrease blood levels.
Tetracyclines, indomethacin, and methyldopa may
increase lithium blood levels.
Haloperidol - Once thought to be contraindicated with
lithium, is now felt to be safe.
Chlorpromazine may increase the rate of lithium excretion.
Tricyclic antidepressants may act synergistically with
lithium.
Aminophylline increases lithium excretion.
Lithium probably prolongs the neuromuscular blocking
effect of succinylcholine.

TREATMENT PRINCIPLES:

- Select appropriate patients. Screen for serious medical
  illness. Pre-administration laboratory evaluation
  should include:

      CBC, BUN, UA
      serum creatinine.
      T3, T4; examine thyroid.

      Serum Na if there is reason to question the
      patient's electrolyte status.
      EKG if the physical or history suggest cardiac
      disease.
      If chronic use of lithium is expected, obtain 24-
      hour urine volume, creatinine clearance, and
      protein excretion.

- Treatment of acute mania:

      The goal is to produce a therapeutic blood level
  (1.2-1.4 meq/l) and maintain it until a clinical
  effect is seen (usually 7-10 days after an appropriate
  level is attained). Begin lithium 300 mg PO BID-TID.
  Always give in divided doses (usually TID-QID).
  Increase by 300 mg every 2-3 days (typical effective
  oral dose is 1200-2400 mg/day).

      Methods to determine the appropriate steady state
  dose of Li based on blood levels following a single
  initial test dose of Li have been developed. As yet,
  none can be considered standard (see Naiman et al,
  1981), but some appear promising (Norman et al, 1982;
  Perry et al, 1982). The ability to quickly select the
  best oral dose of lithium would speed up treatment of
  manic patients markedly.

      Since the mania is not controlled by lithium for
  2-3 weeks, usually also begin an antipsychotic on the
  first day of treatment. Appropriate choices include
  chlorpromazine (300-1200 mg/day or more, in divided
  doses). The antipsychotic provides rapid control of
  the psychomotor activity while the lithium acts more
  gradually but is more specific for control of the
  affect and ideation of mania.

      Once the mania begins to remit, the blood level
  may increase unless the oral dose is reduced. Maintain a therapeutic level until the mania is completely
  controlled (measure blood levels every 1-2 weeks).

- Maintenance treatment of mania:

     If a patient has a history of recurrent mania,
     continue lithium after the acute attack. An effective
     maintenance blood level is 0.5-1.0 meq/l. When stable,
     measure the blood level every 2-3 months.

     Teach the patient to be alert to side effects
     which suggest toxicity - measure lithium level if they
     occur. Lithium level increases with sodium loss so
     advise the patient to be aware of changes in dietary
     salt intake, sweating, and hot climates (although Li
     may be lost more rapidly than sodium, causing the Li
     level to fall - see Jefferson et al, 1982).

     In light of growing evidence of lithium-induced
     renal toxicity, monitor renal function carefully (eg,
     serum creatinine, UA, BUN, protein excretion, and 24-
     hour urine volume every 6-12 months). Also monitor
     thyroid function (eg, T3, T4, and physical examination
     every 6 months).

- If a patient on maintenance lithium shows early signs of
  developing mania, raise the lithium to an acute
  therapeutic level. If the patient develops a
  depression, begin a tricyclic antidepressant.

ANTIDEPRESSANT DRUGS

     The two classes of antidepressant drugs are tricyclic
antidepressants (TCAs) and related drugs and monoamine
oxidase inhibitors (MAOIs). The TCAs are generally the
first choice in treating depressions but the MAOIs have
some specific indications (see below). Lithium carbonate
has a role in treating some major depressions and the
antipsychotic drugs are essential in managing patients with
psychotic depressions.

TRICYCLIC ANTIDEPRESSANTS (TCAs)

DRUGS AVAILABLE: in USA.

TCAs:	Dose (mg/day)
amitriptyline (Elavil, Endep)	75 - 300
amoxapine (Asendin)	100 - 300
desipramine (Norpramin, Pertofrane)	75 - 300
doxepin (Sinequan, Adapin)	75 - 300
imipramine (Tofranil, Presamine)	75 - 300
nortriptyline (Aventyl, Pamelor)	40 - 150

```
protriptyline (Vivactil)                    20 -  60
trimipramine (Surmontil)                    75 - 200
```

Other drugs:

```
maprotiline (Ludiomil)                     100 - 300
trazodone (Desyrel)                        100 - 600
```

INDICATIONS FOR USE:

Recommended for:

1. Major depression - particularly with vegetative
   symptoms and a diurnal variation (70-75% of
   patients respond). TCAs given alone are much less
   successful if there are also psychotic manifestations (eg, hallucinations, delusions, paranoia).
2. Bipolar disorder, depressed or mixed - particularly
   if there are vegetative symptoms. Lithium may be
   useful as well.
3. Short-term maintenance therapy in patients with
   resolved major depression or bipolar disease.
4. Prophylaxis in patients with severe, recurrent
   major depression.
5. Psychotic depression - used concurrently with
   antipsychotics (although ECT is felt by many to
   be the treatment of choice for this condition).
6. Post-partum depressions which are severe.

Other uses:

- Dysthymic disorder - mild chronic depressions
  deserve a trial of TCAs.
- Atypical depression - particularly patients with
  significant anxiety, hypochondriasis, and
  "neurotic" complaints. However, MAOIs may be the
  first choice.
- Panic disorder - may be the treatment of choice but
  the answer is not yet in.
- Agoraphobia - particularly with panic attacks. May
  respond to doses as low as 25 mg/day.
- Obsessive compulsive disorder - particularly those
  patients who also have a depressed mood.
- Childhood conditions - both enuresis and school
  phobia may respond to low doses of a TCA.

TCAs should not be used routinely in the various minor
depressive syndromes.

MECHANISMS OF ACTION:

The effects of TCAs on CNS neurotransmitters are complex and vary from one tricyclic to another. Their therapeutic effects are thought to be related to their ability to increase the amount of CNS interneuronal norepinephrine and serotonin by blocking NE and 5-HT reuptake at the presynaptic membrane. Although affecting both systems, secondary amines (desipramine, protriptyline, and nortriptyline) tend to block NE while tertiary amines (amitriptyline, imipramine, and doxepin) tend to block serotonin - a fact which may account for their observed interpatient response differences.

This growing understanding may be important clinically as there appear to be at least two biochemically distinct types of major depressions which require different anti-depressants. Some depressed patients have low urinary MHPG (a metabolite of NE) and respond to imipramine but not to amitriptyline while other patients have normal or high MHPG levels and respond to amitriptyline but not to imipramine. Conversely, some patients have low CSF 5-HIAA (a metabolite of serotonin) and respond to amitriptyline while others have normal 5-HIAA and improve with imipramine. Currently, use of these biological indicators is still experimental yet they have provided ample justification for trying a second TCA after failure of the first.

PHARMACOKINETICS:

TCAs are absorbed rapidly and completely from the GI tract with peak plasma levels in 1-8 hrs. TCAs are highly bound to plasma and tissue proteins and are fat-soluble - free TCA is only about 1% of the total body load. They are metabolized by the liver and are excreted by the kidney. The half-life ranges from several hours to more than two days.

Do not measure plasma levels routinely, but there are some current indications:

1. Treatment failure - Interindividual plasma levels vary markedly following the same oral dose (10 fold differences) so always consider an ineffective plasma level when explaining a treatment failure. Therapeutic range is 180-225 ng/ml, or higher (or imipramine plus its metabolite, desipramine).

2. Therapeutic window - Some TCAs may have a therapeutic window (eg, nortriptyline and protriptyline are effective primarily at plasma levels of 50-150 ng/ml) while others seem to have no therapeutic upper limit (eg, imipramine).

3. Levels are useful if patient compliance is questioned.
4. Patients with significant side effects may have an excessively high plasma level on a usual oral dosage - measure.
5. Maintain a low plasma level in patients with cardiac disease.
6. Levels are mandatory in serious overdoses.

SIDE EFFECTS:

   Side effects are frequent and usually mild but they can be serious or fatal (particularly cardiac effects in TCA overdoses) and are more common in the elderly.

   Anticholinergic:
      dry mouth
      blurred vision (near vision)
      constipation, urinary hesitancy

   Autonomic:
      tremor (fine, rapid, usually hands and fingers)
      sweating
      impotence, ejaculatory dysfunction

   Cardiac:
      In normal dosages:
         orthostatic hypotension, tachycardia.
         EKG changes (T-wave flattening, increased PR and QT interval).
      In overdose:
         PVCs, ventricular arrhythmias
         AV block and BBB.
         CHF and cardiac arrest.

   Other:
      sedation
      restlessness, insomnia
      rashes, allergic reactions
      wt gain
      anorexia, nausea and vomiting
      EEG changes
      confusion (in elderly)
      seizures in patients who are predisposed

   Tolerance usually develops to the anticholinergic and sedative side effects. Use cautiously in the elderly and in patients with BPH - avoid in patients with narrow-angle glaucoma. Pregnancy is not a contraindication for TCA use since there is no convincing evidence of teratogenicity, but avoid use in the first trimester if possible.

Most worrisome are the cardiac effects. There have been a few reports of sudden death from presumed arrhythmias - patients with pre-existing heart disease (particularly bundle-branch disease) and/or hypertension (eg, the elderly) are at risk for any of the cardiac side effects. Do not use following an acute MI or while in CHF. The danger is greatest with higher doses - eg, following an OD with a TCA.

There are wide differences between agents in their ability to produce some side effects and these should be considered when choosing a drug. The presence of side effects is not a good indication that a therapeutic plasma level has been reached.

Tricyclic	Anticholinergic	Sedation
amitriptyline	5+	5+
amoxapine	2+	2+
desipramine	1+	1+
doxepin	3+	5+
imipramine	4+	3+
maprotiline	2+	3+
nortriptyline	3+	2+
protriptyline	3+	1+
trazadone	1+	2+
trimipramine	2+	4+

Certain psychiatric conditions may be adversely affected by TCAs.

- Schizophrenia may be made worse.
- A depressed bipolar patient may become manic.

A withdrawal syndrome occurs in some patients who have been taking high doses of TCAs (eg, imipramine 150-300 mg/day) for weeks or months. If medication is stopped abruptly, symptoms begin in 1-2 days and include anxiety, headache, myalgia, chills, malaise, and nausea. Withdraw the medication gradually (eg, 25-50 mg/wk).

Several new, non-tricyclic antidepressants are now available which are reputed to have an efficacy equal to or greater than the TCAs but with fewer side effects: maprotiline, amoxapine, trazodone. Moreover, others are "waiting in the wings" for release. Although some (eg, trazodone) are almost side effect-free (mild headache, lethargy, nausea), clear indications for use await further experience. Unwanted side effects have appeared with some - eg, grand mal seizures (maprotiline) and painful and/or retrograde ejaculation (amoxapine).

DRUG INTERACTIONS:

- TCA plasma level is increased (at times dangerously) by methylphenidate, Antabuse, antipsychotics, exogenous thyroid, and guanethidine.
- TCA plasma level is decreased (frequently below therapeutic range) by barbiturates, alcohol, and smoking (may need to monitor level in heavy smokers).
- CNS depression occurs with antipsychotics, hypnotic-sedatives, anticonvulsants, and alcohol.
- TCAs impair the antihypertensive effect of methyldopa, guanethidine, and bethanidine.
- There is a synergistic anticholinergic effect with other central anticholinergics - may produce a toxic psychosis.
- Marked hypertension can be caused by administration of TCAs with sympathomimetic drugs (eg, isoproterenol, epinephrine, phenylephrine, amphetamines).
- TCAs may dangerously increase the half-life of anti-coagulants (eg, Dicumarol) - monitor prothrombin time.

TREATMENT PRINCIPLES:

- Identify the patient likely to benefit from a TCA.
    1. Appropriate clinical presentation.
    2. Past personal history of good TCA response.
    3. Past family history of good TCA response.
    4. If available, urinary MHPG levels may point toward an appropriate TCA (Cobbin, et al, 1979).

- Unless side effects are likely to be a problem, begin with a tertiary TCA. They are metabolized in the liver to secondary TCAs (imipramine to desipramine; amitriptyline to nortriptyline) and thus both the tertiary and secondary TCAs are present in the body. However, these rules may change as we learn more about the indications for the newer antidepressants such as trazodone.

- Side effects may be useful (eg, use sedating amitriptyline for an agitated depression; use desipramine for those elderly who are sensitive to anticholinergic side effects).

- One technique for treating depression with TCAs is:

    Begin imipramine 50 mg PO HS (or equivalent - less in elderly; more in the obese) and increase by 25 mg every 2-3 days until 150 mg is reached. If side effects interfere, slow down.
    Hold dosage at 150 mg for 1 week, then, if depression

remains, increase in 25 mg steps to 200 mg (50 mg during the day, 150 mg at HS).
Hold dosage at 200 mg for one week, then increase in 25 mg steps to 300 mg (150 mg in divided doses during the day, 150 mg at HS). Consider hospitalizing the patient for trials above 200 mg/day. Maintain at 300 mg for 2-3 weeks. If depression remains:
1. Has patient been taking medication?
2. Has a therapeutic window been passed?
3. Measure plasma level.
If the patient is unimproved, consider:
1. A different TCA.
2. ECT.
3. An MAOI. Allow 1-2 wks for transfer.
With a good response, sleep and appetite usually return first, then an improved mood. There is usually a 1-3 wk delay in the therapeutic effect so don't stop meds prematurely.

- Never give a worrisomely depressed or seriously suicidal patient a prescription for more than 1000 mg of imipramine (or equivalent).

- If treating a psychotic depression, use a TCA and an antipsychotic simultaneously.

- If treating a depression in a bipolar patient taking lithium, continue the lithium if it has been effective prophylactically. The lithium may help prevent a manic overshoot.

- If treating a phobic-anxiety disorder, expect improvement with a lower dosage (eg, 100 mg).

- Simultaneous use of a TCA and an MAOI is currently discouraged by the FDA, but is often useful.

- Maintenance care: In a successfully treated patient, wait 2 months, then decrease the medication by 25 mg/wk until at one half the therapeutic dose. Wait 2-4 months. If the patient has had several recurrences of a major depression in the past, consider long-term TCA maintenance (reduces likelihood of a relapse by 50%). Consider lithium maintenance in a recurrent bipolar illness. If there is no previous history of illness, gradually withdraw the medication.

- TCA overdose is life-threatening and should be treated on a medical inpatient unit. Recognize that dangerously high plasma levels may continue for more than one week.

- Although generally not considered drugs of abuse, a recent report (Cohn et al, 1978) describes significant illicit use of amitriptyline by an outpatient population of narcotic abusers. Watch for it.

MONOAMINE OXIDASE INHIBITORS (MAOIs)

DRUGS AVAILABLE:

Drug	Dose (mg/day)
HYDRAZIDE MAOIs	
phenelzine (Nardil)	45 - 90
isocarboxazid (Marplan)	10 - 30
NONHYDRAZIDE MAOIs	
tranylcypromine (Parnate)	10 - 60

INDICATIONS FOR USE:

Recommended for:

1. Atypical depression - MAOIs should probably be the drug of choice for "atypical, neurotic depressions" (50-60% improve) - ie, patients with varying degrees of depressive and anxious affect, rejection sensitivity, irritability, emotional lability, hyperphagia, hypersomnolence, reversed diurnal variation (worse in evening), and hypochondriasis (all with the vegetative symptoms of a major depression). If a TCA is tried first and fails, follow with a trial of an MAOI. ECT is notoriously unsuccessful with these patients.

Other uses:

- Patients with major depression or dysthymic disorder who have not improved with a trial of one or more TCA and for whom ECT is not the obvious next choice. Has the patient or a family member responded to an MAOI in the past?
- Although not approved by the FDA, MAOIs appear useful in panic disorder and in agoraphobia with panic attacks.
- Certain MAOIs (eg, clorgyline) may be useful for rapid-cycling affective disorder (four or more episodes/yr).

MECHANISMS OF ACTION:

MAOIs block MAO (and other enzymes) throughout the body (eg, blood, platelets, gut, CNS). MAO catalyzes the oxidation of the biogenic amines tyramine, 5-HT, DA, and NE. The therapeutic effect of MAOIs is <u>probably</u> related to the increase in CNS NE and 5-HT which results from the ability of MAOI to block this oxidation of intracellular catecholamines.

MAO apparently exists in two forms: type A (MAO-A) which acts primarily on 5-HT and NE, and type B (MAO-B) which acts on DA and phenylethylamine. They both act on tyramine. The MAOIs phenelzine and tranylcypromine inhibit both types of MAO, clorgyline (not on the market - see Potter et al, 1982) inhibits MAO-A, while pargyline (Eutonyl - used as an antihypertensive, not an antidepressant) inhibits MAO-B. MAO-A inhibitors may be more effective antidepressants, while MAO-B inhibitors are less prone to produce hypertensive reactions. More work remains to be done.

PHARMACOKINETICS:

MAOIs are rapidly absorbed and are metabolized into inactive products by several means including acetylation (hydrazide MAOIs only). There may be patients who are "rapid acetylators" and who require increased oral doses of MAOI for improvement to occur. There is usually a delay of 1-4 weeks before a clinical response is seen. Measured inhibition of platelet MAO in blood samples (80-90% inhibition appears necessary) provides some indication that an effective level of CNS MAOI has been reached, although this procedure is currently primarily a research technique.

SIDE EFFECTS:

MAOIs have fewer side effects than TCAs and are often better tolerated by patients. They do not have the range of cardiotoxic effects of the TCAs although some experts feel that they should be contraindicated in the elderly because of the risk of hypertensive crisis (see below) with its potentially fatal outcome in the older patient.

The most common side effects include drowsiness or stimulation (short lived), <u>insomnia</u>, giddiness, dizziness, dry mouth, impotence, orthostatic <u>hypotension</u>, constipation, and weight gain. They also can precipitate a manic or schizoaffective attack. Since occasional patients develop hepatotoxicity, patients using MAOIs long-term should have periodic examinations of liver function. They are contraindicated in patients with liver disease, CHF, or pheochromocytoma.

The most serious (but infrequent - see Folks, 1983) side effect is hypertension (hypertensive crisis, cerebrovascular bleeding) and hyperpyrexia in response to ingested tyramine (or other pressor amines). The MAO in the gut wall which usually prevents entrance of large quantities of ingested pressor amines is inhibited by MAOIs, thus allowing a generalized sympathetic effect when tyramine-containing foods are eaten. The first sign of an impending crisis is usually a sudden, severe occipital or temporal headache (also sweating, fever, neck stiffness, photophobia). Patients taking MAOIs should avoid:

    Protein-containing foods which are cultured or spoiled:
        Pickled or kippered herring; dried, salted fish.
        Chicken livers or liver pate; any slightly spoiled
            meat; ripened sausages.
        Nondistilled alcohol - red or Chianti wine; beer.
        Strong cheeses (cottage, ricotta, or cream cheese are
            OK).
        Old yogurt, chocolate.

    Broad beans (Fava, Italian Green, and Lima beans).

A number of adrenergic drugs (see below) may also produce a hypertensive crisis. If one occurs, treat with slow administration of phentolamine (Regitine, 5 mg IV). It usually resolves in a few hours. The patient may carry one dose of 50 mg phentolamine with him with instructions to take it orally when signs of a crisis appear.

DRUG INTERACTIONS:

    Hypertensive crisis - can be produced by amphetamines,
        cocaine, and anorectics (stimulate NE release from
        adrenergic neurons), catecholamines (epinephrine, NE),
        sympathomimetic precursors (dopamine, methyldopa,
        levodopa), and sympathomimetic amines (ephedrine,
        phenylephrine, phenylpropanolamine, pseudoephedrine,
        metaraminol, over-the-counter cold and hay fever
        medication).
    Meperidine (Demerol) - A few patients develop severe,
        immediate hypertension and sweating or hypotension and
        coma. Narcotics may act similarly.
    CNS depression - potentiated by alcohol, hypnotic-
        sedatives, and major tranquilizers.
    Concurrent use of MAOIs and TCAs may increase the risk of
        a hypertensive crisis. This combination is not
        approved by the FDA but may be useful for some
        patients.

TREATMENT PRINCIPLES:

- Instruct the patient carefully about the potential side effects and the drugs and foods to avoid.

- Begin phenelzine 15 mg PO BID-TID and increase by 15 mg weekly to 60-90 mg/day. Maintain that dosage for 4-6 weeks before assuming a failure.

- Maintenance is at one half maximum dose (similar to TCAs). In some patients, for unknown reasons, both the antidepressant and antiphobic effects become ineffective after 6 months to one year of use.

- Allow for a one week washout before starting another medication.

- If insomnia becomes a major problem, give all doses before midafternoon.

- Recognize that a few patients may require an MAOI and TCA combination if they are to improve.

- Tranylcypromine (1) has significant stimulant properties and (2) may be more effective in major depression than other MAOIs. It also produces a more rapid onset of clinical effects.

- Don't give impulsive, potentially suicidal outpatients large prescriptions.

ANTIANXIETY AGENTS

DRUGS AVAILABLE:

There are numerous drugs available for sedation, of which only the benzodiazepines can be recommended.

Drug	Half-life (hrs)	Dose (mg/day)
alprazolam (Xanax)	11-14	2-4
chlorazepate (Tranxene)	30-65	15-60
chlordiazepoxide (Librium)	24-48	15-100
diazepam (Valium)	20-50	5-30
lorazepam (Ativan)	9-12	2-10
oxazepam (Serax)	3-21	30-120
flurazepam (Dalmane)	3-8	15-30 (HS)
temazepam (Restoril)	5-15	15-30 (HS)
triazolam (Halcion)	2-3	0.125-0.5(HS)

INDICATIONS FOR USE:

1. Short-term treatment of restlessness and anxiety (eg, following life crises). They are sedative at low dosage and hypnotic at higher doses. They have no antipsychotic activity and thus should not be used as the exclusive treatment for psychotic disorders.
2. Alcohol withdrawal (see chapter 16).
3. Various seizure disorders.
4. Muscle relaxant (diazepam).

MECHANISMS OF ACTION AND PHARMACOKINETICS:

They enhance the inhibitory neurotransmitters (eg, GABA, glycine) and they have a specific depressant effect on the limbic system. As the dosage rises, there is generalized CNS depression.

They are well absorbed orally, are all both water and lipid soluble, and are usually metabolized by the liver but may also be excreted by the kidney. They are slowly and variably absorbed IM (faster by PO route). There is very little hepatic enzyme induction. Peak blood levels usually occur 1-4 hours after the oral dose.

SIDE EFFECTS

In comparison to other classes of psychoactive drugs, side effects are few.

- Most common problem is CNS depression manifested by daytime sedation, decreased concentration, and poor coordination in some patients at therapeutic doses. They are very safe drugs although a massive OD will produce life-threatening CNS depression.
- Anterograde amnesia is common following hypnotic-induced sleep. Patients may lose memory for events which occurred during the night or during the following day (Shader and Greenblatt, 1983).
- Tolerance and physical addiction are unusual but do occur at high doses when taken for several months. The withdrawal syndrome is usually mild (but may be severe) and typically occurs 4-14 days after stopping the drug.
- Untoward but infrequent psychiatric manifestations include exacerbation of schizophrenia and depression.
- There appear to be no autonomic side effects.

DRUG INTERACTIONS

There is an increased sedative effect when combined with CNS depressants (eg, alcohol). Moreover, the combina-

tion with alcohol at times actually may be anxiogenic.
Disulfiram (Antabuse) impairs the metabolism of the long-
acting benzodiazepines and thus raises the plasma
levels. The shorter-acting drugs appear less affected.
Food and antacids appear to decrease the rate but not the
extent of drug absorption.

TREATMENT PRINCIPLES:

- Use the long-acting benzodiazepines (chlordiazepoxide,
  diazepam) on an HS or BID schedule. Use a TID-QID
  schedule for the shorter-acting ones (oxazepam,
  lorazepam).
- Recognize that the longer-acting drugs may accumulate
  over days or weeks, producing increasing symptoms of
  sedation, etc. Lorazepam and oxazepam do not
  accumulate.
- Do not use longer than 1-3 weeks in most patients either
  as a sedative or a hypnotic. Some patients may be
  able to use less frequently but long-term on an "as
  needed" basis but be alert for those patients prone to
  abuse.
- Use by PO route, if possible.
- Encourage the patient to avoid the simultaneous use of a
  benzodiazepine and alcohol or another sedative-hypnotic
  drug. Do not prescribe more than a 2 weeks' supply at
  any one time.
- Be very careful when giving to the elderly - confusion is
  common.
- Several of these drugs are preferred as hypnotics
  (usually because of shorter half-lives and less REM
  suppression). Flurazepam and triazolam (short half-
  life) are useful for sleep onset problems; temazepam
  and flurazepam may help frequent awakening.

ELECTROCONVULSIVE THERAPY (ECT)

In spite of its notoriety, ECT is a legitimate
psychiatric treatment. Although its mechanism of action is
unknown, it is effective, painless, and safe, with a
mortality rate (.01-.03% of patients treated - mostly
cardiovascular deaths) less than competing therapies or the
untreated state. However, because of its legal
sensitivity, prior to administration always obtain:

1. Informed consent from a voluntary, competent patient.
2. Informed consent from a relative or guardian of a
     voluntary, incompetent patient and an independent
     psychiatric opinion of therapeutic need.
3. Court approval for administration to a resisting,

involuntary patient who is a danger to himself or
others.

Discuss the risks of amnesia, confusion, and headache with
the patient and his family. Also discuss the risks of not
receiving ECT.

Indications for use:

ECT is a serious procedure - use only in those
conditions for which it is recommended. It is tempting to
give ECT to any patient who is not improving - don't!

MAJOR AFFECTIVE ILLNESS: Patients with Major Depression
or Bipolar disorder, depressed respond well to ECT
(80-90% recover vs 60-70% treated with antidepressants).
Patients with marked vegetative symptoms (eg, insomnia,
constipation, suicidal ruminations, obsessions with
guilt, anorexia and wt loss, psychomotor retardation)
are particularly responsive. ECT is much more
effective than antidepressants for psychotically
depressed patients - ie, vegetative symptoms and
paranoid or somatic delusions. Give antidepressants a
full trial (eg, imipramine 200-300 mg/day for 3 weeks),
then consider ECT if there is no improvement.
Mania (Bipolar Disorder, manic) also responds to
ECT but it should be used only if lithium carbonate
(often initially coupled with an antipsychotic) fails
to control the acute phase.

SCHIZOPHRENIC DISORDERS: Catatonic Schizophrenia of
either stuporous or excited type responds well to ECT.
Try antipsychotic medication first but, if the
condition is life-threatening (eg, hyperexcited
delirium), go quickly to ECT. An occasional acutely
psychotic patient (particularly of the schizoaffective
type) who does not respond to medication may improve
with ECT, but for most schizophrenics (eg, chronics) it
is of little value.

ECT is the treatment of choice for:

1. Actively suicidal depressed patients who may not
   live until antidepressants begin to work.
2. Depressed patients (particularly the elderly) whose
   medical condition makes administration of antidepressants risky. Patients with both depression
   and OBS may do better with ECT. ECT can be safely
   performed during pregnancy.
3. Seriously depressed patients who have had an
   adequate trial of antidepressants (60-70% recover
   with ECT).

Contraindications for use:

There are no absolute contraindications. Always weigh
the risk of the procedure against the danger incurred if
the patient is untreated. Response improves with age -
patients under 30 respond poorly.

Very high risk:
Increased intracranial pressure (eg, brain tumor, CNS
infection): ECT briefly increases CSF pressure and
risks tentorial herniation. Always check for
papilledema before administration.
Recent MI: ECT frequently causes arrhythmias (vagal
arrhythmias producing postictal PVCs and extravagal
arrhythmias producing PVCs anytime during the
procedure) which can be fatal if there has been
recent muscle damage. Wait until enzymes and EKG
have stabilized.

Moderate risk:
Severe osteoarthritis, osteoporosis, or recent
fracture: Prepare thoroughly for treatment (ie,
with muscle relaxants).
Cardiovascular disease (eg, hypertension, angina,
aneurysm, arrhythmias): Premedicate carefully;
have a cardiologist available.
Major infections, recent CVA, chronic respiratory
difficulty, acute peptic ulcer.

TECHNIQUE OF ADMINISTRATION:

Pre-ECT Medical Workup:

Complete history and physical concentrating on cardiac
and neurological status, CBC, chemistry, UA, VDRL, chest
and spine X-rays, EKG. Get EEG (and/or CT scan) if
neurological is abnormal.

A Typical Technique:

ECT routines vary - there is no "one right way."
Usually perform in a hospital and with the aid of an
anesthesiologist.

1. Prepare the patient with information and psychological
support. Have him void and defecate beforehand. NPO
after midnight. If markedly anxious, give 5 mg of
diazepam IM 1-2 hrs before treatment. Antidepressants
and antipsychotics should be stopped the day before
treatment. Lithium and ECT may be given concurrently
if cardiac and renal functions are good.

2. Make patient comfortable. Remove dentures. Hyperextend the back with a pillow.
3. When ready, premedicate with atropine (0.6-1.2 mg SC, IM, or IV). This anticholinergic controls vagal arrhythmias and reduces GI secretions.
4. Provide 90-100% oxygen by bag when respirations are not spontaneous.
5. Give sodium methohexital (Brevital) (40-100 mg IV, rapidly). This short-acting barbiturate anesthetic is used to produce a light coma.
6. Next quickly give enough of the muscle relaxant succinylcholine (Anectine) (30-80 mg IV, rapidly - monitor depth of relaxation by the muscle fascicula- tions produced) to remove all but very minor evidences of a generalized seizure (eg, plantarflexion).
7. Once relaxed, place a bite-block in the mouth and then give electroconvulsive stimulus. Two methods are common today:

> Unilateral: One electrode placed in the frontotemporal area and the other 7-10 cm away in the parietal region - both on the nondominant hemisphere (right side for right-handed persons, 60% R and 40% L for left-handers). Unilateral ECT produces less postictal confusion and amnesia but may be slightly less effective. It is usually the method of choice.
> Bilateral: Bifrontotemporal electrode placement. This is the traditional technique - effective but produces more side effects (eg, amnesia, headache).

> Effectiveness of either method depends upon producing a central generalized seizure (peripheral effects are not necessary) lasting at least 25 seconds. Monitor this with EEG, peripheral EMG, or the tonic/clonic movement of the hand on the same side as the electrode (unilateral) which has been freed of muscle relaxant by a tight cuff applied before the administration of the succinylcholine. If a seizure is not produced, increase the stimulus and repeat ("missed" or unilateral seizures are usually of little therapeutic value - they occur more frequently with unilateral shock, perhaps accounting for its lesser effectiveness).

8. Monitor patient carefully until stable - there is usually 15-30 minutes of postictal confusion. These patients are at risk for prolonged apnea and a postictal delirium (5-10 mg of IV diazepam may help).

Complications of ECT:

- Amnesia (retrograde and anterograde) - variable;

> beginning after 3-4 treatments; lasting weeks to 2-3
> months (but occasionally much longer); more severe
> with bilateral placement, increased number of
> treatments, and increased current strength.
- Headache, muscle aches, nausea.
- Dizziness, confusion - The persistence and severity of
  the confusion increases with an increasing number of
  treatments.
- Reserpine and ECT given concurrently have resulted in
  fatalities.
- Fractures - rare with good muscle relaxation.
- ECT anesthesia risks:
  Atropine worsens narrow angle glaucoma.
  Succinylcholine's action is prolonged in pseudo-
      cholinesterase deficiency states. These conditions
      (malnutrition, liver disease, chronic renal
      dialysis, use of echothiophate for glaucoma) can
      lead to potentially fatal hypotonia. Procainamide,
      lidocaine, and quinidine can potentiate succinyl-
      choline.
  Methohexital can precipitate an attack of acute
      intermittent porphyria.

Treatment Principles:

1. Usually give one treatment/day - on alternate days.
2. Depressions usually require 6-12 treatments. Mania and
   catatonia require 10-20. Expect to see improved
   behavior after 2-6 treatments if it is going to be
   effective. Allow the clinical response to determine
   the treatment endpoint. Be very cautious (and seek a
   second opinion) about exceeding 20 treatments during
   one period of illness.
3. Maintenance ECT (single treatments every 4-6 weeks
   during the months or years after recovery) may be
   useful, particularly with elderly depressed patients,
   but should be used only if medication is contraindicated.
4. Maintenance antidepressants, antipsychotics, and lithium
   (begin after a successful course of ECT) definitely
   forestall relapse. Without medication, the relapse
   rate is high.

PSYCHOSURGERY

Little psychosurgery is currently performed in the
USA. Modern psychosurgeons make one of several possible
small cuts in the brain (usually in the limbic system)
which can improve a variety of psychiatric conditions and
which have few side effects (unlike the widely destructive
prefrontal lobotomy of the past).

All candidates for surgery must have an intractable and devastating condition unrelieved by any other therapy. Conditions likely to respond include chronic pain with depression and severe depression alone. Improvement occurs in some patients who have severe obsessive-compulsive and anxiety states and in a few schizophrenics. The mechanism for the improvement is unknown and a variety of different "cuts" yield similar results. Despite the lack of theoretical sophistication, there are patients for whom psychosurgery is a valid "last resort."

REFERENCES

1. American Psychiatric Association: Electroconvulsive Therapy. Task Force Report 14. Wash., DC, 1978.
2. Amsterdam J, Brunswick D, Mendels J: The clinical application of tricyclic antidepressant pharmacokinetics and plasma levels. Am J Psychiat 137:643, 1980.
3. Branchey M, Branchey L: Patterns of psychotropic drug use and tardive dyskinesia. J Clin Psychopharm 4:41, 1984.
4. Caroff SN: The neuroleptic malignant syndrome. J Clin Psychiat 41:79, March, 1980.
5. Cobbin DM, Requin-Blow B, Williams LR, Williams WO: Urinary MHPG levels and tricyclic antidepressant drug selection. Arch Gen Psychiat 36:1111, 1979.
6. Cohen MJ, Hanbury R, Stimmel B: Abuse of amitriptyline. JAMA 240:1372, 1978.
7. Cohen S: A clinical appraisal of diazepam. Psychosomatics 22:761, 1981.
8. Delva NJ, Letemendia FJJ: Lithium treatment in schizophrenia and schizo-affective disorders. Brit J Psychiat 141:387, 1982.
9. Fink M: Convulsive Therapy: Theory and Practice. New York, Raven Pr, 1979.
10. Folks DG: Monoamine oxidase inhibitors: reappraisal of dietary considerations. J Clin Psychopharm 3:249, 1983.
11. Glassman AH, Bigger JT: Cardiovascular effects of therapeutic doses of tricyclic antidepressants. Arch Gen Psychiat 38:815, 1981.
12. Granacher RP: Differential diagnosis of tardive dyskinesia: an overview. Am J Psychiat 138:1288, 1981.
13. Granacher RP, Baldessarini RJ: Physostigmine: its use in acute anticholinergic syndrome with antidepressant and antiparkinson drugs. Arch Gen Psychiat 32:375, 1975.
14. Jefferson JW, Greist JH, Clagnaz PJ, Eischens RR, Marten WC, Evenson MA: Effect of strenuous exercise on serum lithium level in man. Am J Psychiat 139:1593, 1982.

15. Kane JM, Rifkin A, Woerner M, Reardon G, Sarantakos S, Schiebel D, Ramos-Lorenzi J: Low-dose neuroleptic treatment of outpatient schizophrenics. Arch Gen Psychiat 40:893, 1983.
16. Kane JM, Smith JM: Tardive Dyskinesia: prevalence and risk factors. Arch Gen Psychiat 39:473, 1982.
17. Keepers GA, Clappison VJ, Casey DE: Initial anticholinergic prophylaxis for neuroleptic-induced extrapyramidal syndromes. Arch Gen Psychiat 40:1113, 1983.
18. Lipton MA, DiMascio A, Killam KF: Psychopharmacology: A Generation of Progress. New York, Raven Pr, 1978.
19. McEvoy: The clinical use of anticholinergic drugs as treatment for extrapyramidal side effects of neuroleptic drugs. J Clin Psychopharm 3:288, 1983.
20. Mitchell JE, Popkin MK: Antidepressant drug therapy and sexual dysfunction in men: a review. J Clin Psychopharm 3:76, 1983.
21. Mueller PS, Vester JW, Fermaglich J: Neuroleptic malignant syndrome: successful treatment with bromocriptine. JAMA 249:386, 1983.
22. Naiman IF, Muniz CE, Stewart RB, Yost RL: Practicality of a lithium dosing guide. Am J Psychiat 138:1369, 1981.
23. Norman KP, Cerrone KL, Reus VI: Renal lithium clearance as a rapid and accurate predictor of maintenance dose. Am J Psychiat 139:1625, 1982.
24. Perry PJ, Alexander B, Dunner FJ, Schoenwald RD, Pfohl B, Miller D: Pharmacokinetic protocol for predicting serum lithium levels. J Clin Psychopharm 2:114, 1982.
25. Potter WZ, Murphy DL, Wehr TA, Linnoila M, Goodwin FK: Clorgyline. Arch Gen Psychiat 39:505, 1982.
26. Quitkin F, Rifkin A, Klein DF: Monoamine oxidase inhibitors: a review of antidepressant effectiveness. Arch Gen Psychiat 36:749, 1979.
27. Ramsey TA, Cox M: Lithium and the kidney: a review. Am J Psychiat 139:443, 1982.
28. Scovern AW, Kilmann PR: Status of electroconvulsive therapy: review of the outcome literature. Psycho Bull 87:260, 1980.
29. Shader RI, Greenblatt DJ: Editorial: triazolam and anterograde amnesia. J Clin Psychopharm 3:273, 1983.
30. Squire LR, Slater PC: Electroconvulsive therapy and complaints of memory dysfunction: a prospective three-year follow-up study. Brit J Psychiat 142:1, 1983.
31. Stern SL, Rush AJ, Mendels J: Toward a rational pharmacotherapy of depression. Am J Psychiat 137:545, 1980.
32. Tarsy D: Neuroleptic-induced extrapyramidal reactions: classification, description, and diagnosis. Clin Neuropharm 6: Suppl 1, S9, 1983.

33. Todd R, Lippmann S, Manshadi M, Chang A: Recognition
    and treatment of rabbit syndrome, an uncommon
    complication of neuroleptic therapies. Am J Psychiat
    140:1519, 1983.
34. Tyrer P, Gardner M, Lambourn J, Whitford M: Clinic and
    pharmacokinetic factors affecting response to
    phenelzine. Brit J Psychiat 136:359, 1980.
35. Van Putten T: Vulnerability to extrapyramidal side
    effects. Clin Neuropharm 6: Suppl 1,27, 1983.
36. Van Putten T, May PRA, Marder SR: Response to
    antipsychotic medication: the doctor's and the
    consumer's view. Am J Psychiat 141:16, 1984.

Chapter 24

The Elderly Patient

More than 25,000,000 Americans are over 65. 85% have a chronic illness (usually medical) while only 20-30% have a psychiatric illness (percentage rises as the population gets older).

EVALUATION OF THE ELDERLY

1. Assess each patient carefully - mental decline is <u>not</u> "normal" for the aged.
2. Always carefully evaluate physical condition. An impaired physical state can markedly alter the psychiatric evaluation. Make sure the patient can hear and see. Check for deficiency states (iron, folate, vitamin B_{12} and D, calcium, serum proteins).
3. Interview technique: Be respectful, use surname, sit near, speak slowly and clearly, allow time for answers, be friendly and personal, pat and hug, be supportive and issue-oriented, keep interview short.
4. Collect history, do mental status - perhaps in more than one interview.
5. Identify premorbid personality - defense mechanisms and coping styles (eg, independent vs passive-dependent, rigid vs flexible, use of denial, etc).
6. Assess the major <u>risk factors</u>:
   A. Loss - of spouse, <u>friends</u>, physical health, job, status, independence, etc.
   B. Poverty - many elderly are poor; some are victims of crime.
   C. Social isolation - impaired mobility, few friends, etc.
   D. Sensory deprivation - poor hearing, vision, etc.
   E. Sickness - chronic pain, forced inactivity, etc.
   F. Fears - of being dependent, of being alone, of being helpless.

7. See family - assess their strengths, dynamics, support
   for the patient, hidden agendas.

COMMON PSYCHIATRIC DISORDERS

Delirium (see p 51): Common (Lipowski, 1983). May be the
primary presentation of:
1. CNS - Cerebral infarction (embolic or thrombotic),
   TIA, neoplasms.
2. Heart - MI (often without pain), arrhythmia, CHF.
3. Lungs - Pneumonia (without fever or leukocytosis), PE
   (without chest pain, dyspnea, tachycardia).
4. Blood - Anemia.
5. Metabolic - Diabetes, liver failure, hyper- or
   hypothyroidism, electrolyte abnormalities.
6. Psychogenic - strange surroundings, stress.
7. Infections - most kinds.
8. Other - Medication reaction, alcoholism, prescription
   drug misuse, dehydration, fecal impaction, "silent"
   appendicitis, urinary retention, UTIs, eye or ear
   disease, postoperative.

Treat the underlying disease process, if possible.
Keep patient in a lighted room and with familiar surroundings and people. Restrain only if essential. If needed,
use small doses of major tranquilizers (eg, thioridazine
25-50 mg, PO, often given as an HS dose; thiothixene 2-5
mg, PO, or 4 mg, IM).

Dementia: Most elderly have unimpaired intellectual
functioning. Dementia (20% of those 80 years old) is not
"just a result of aging" - it needs an explanation (see p
57). Dementia often presents first with agitation,
anxiety, depression, and/or somatic complaints - always do
a mental status exam on elderly patients with these
complaints but, remember, that it can also be mimicked by
depression, serious physical conditions, alcoholism, and
malnutrition. Dementia in the elderly frequently occurs
with and is made worse by depression or delirium. The
memory loss is often unrecognized by the patient but is of
major concern to the family, who ultimately insist on
evaluation and treatment for it.

Most patients with a progressive and non-reversible
form of dementia can be maintained at home until the late
stages of the disease process. The decision to institu-
tionalize depends not only on what facilities are available
locally (some may be very good) but also on the realistic
strengths and limits of the family. Once the cause and
prognosis of the dementia is determined, the physician may
most profitably spend his time helping the family adjust.

Depression: Major Depression can develop in old age for the
first time or as a recurrence of a major affective
disorder. In the elderly it may at times closely mimic a
dementia (pseudodementia - see p 62) - or physical
symptoms, apathy, or fatigue may dominate the clinical
picture. Remember that the highest suicide rate occurs
among elderly males (particularly with alcoholism) so, if
in doubt, hospitalize. Treat with psychotherapy and
antidepressants (increase slowly; effective final daily
dose may be as low as 75-100 mg). ECT may be the therapy
of choice in patients with unstable cardiac status or in
those patients with psychotic depression (eg, paranoia,
hallucinations).

A less severe depression or depressive equivalent
(listlessness, physical complaints, withdrawal) in a
patient with longstanding depressive complaints may
represent Dysthymic Disorder (see p 41). Since stress and
loss are so common among the elderly, Adjustment Disorder
with Depressed Mood (see p 42) and Uncomplicated
Bereavement (see p 84) occur frequently.

Mania: Does occur in old age but almost invariably with a
history of bipolar disorder. Extreme agitation or manic-
like behavior can be caused by delirium, dementia,
schizophrenia, depression, or situational anxiety. Lithium
is effective.

Schizophrenia: Usually there is a life-long history of
schizophrenic illness but, rarely, the stresses of old age
can precipitate a first episode in a predisposed individual
(longstanding schizoid or borderline functioning).
Occasionally there is associated intellectual deterioration. Treat with support and antipsychotics.

Paranoia: Mild suspiciousness among the elderly is very
common. Bizarre forms or near psychotic levels may occur
with:

1. Early dementia - always check for intellectual loss.
2. Delirium
3. Vision or hearing problems - may resolve promptly.
4. Social isolation; chronic illness.
5. Drugs - eg, steroids, antiparkinsonians, hypnotic
   withdrawal.

The psychotic disorder, PARANOIA (DSM-III p 197,
297.10), often has an onset late in life (late paraphrenia).
These patients have fixed paranoid delusions and occasionally auditory hallucinations but not the loose associations,
grandiosity, major hallucinations, and autistic thought of
paranoid schizophrenics (although the conditions may

overlap). Treat with reality-oriented psychotherapy, behavior modification, maintenance antipsychotics, and possibly ECT.

Hypochondriasis: The elderly are frequently ill and may develop a preoccupation with exaggerated physical complaints and problems. This is particularly common among depressed and/or demented elderly. The physical symptoms may or may not improve with resolution of the depression.

The patient with severe hypochondriasis, whose life is dominated by ruminations about one or more physical problems, is very difficult to treat. Withdrawal and isolation are frequent. Don't expect a "cure". Develop an ongoing relationship with this patient. Be available. See every 2-3 weeks for 10-20 minutes. Reassure that the problem may be persistent and incurable but not debilitating or fatal. Recognize that in some cases symptoms may continue because to lose them would mean to lose the reason for visiting the physician.

Adjustment Disorders: These are common in old age and are due to the numerous stresses (loss, physical illness, retirement, etc.) encountered. Symptoms include anxiety, depression, agitation, and physical complaints and most often occur in persons with past adjustment problems. Grief is common and may mimic a major depression but often has an obvious precipitant, is short-lived with therapy, and does not require antidepressants. Alcohol abuse is also a common response to stress in the elderly. Supportive psychotherapy, attention to concrete problems, and brief use of minor tranquilizers or low-dose antipsychotics help.

PSYCHOPHARMACOLOGY OF OLD AGE

The elderly usually run higher blood levels (due to decreased hepatic metabolism and renal excretion, reduced plasma albumin and protein binding, and increased fat to lean tissue ratios), display increased receptor responsiveness, and thus require more gradual increases and lower doses of most psychoactive medication. They are also more susceptible to most side effects - eg, peripheral and central anticholinergic effects, sedation, hypotension, arrhythmias. They are at risk for bowel obstruction, urinary retention, BP problems (fainting, stroke), sudden death from fatal arrhythmias, glaucoma crises, delirium, and coma. Also, they are particularly likely to be taking multiple drugs, to misunderstand and fail to comply with prescribing instruction, and to have symptoms from such polypharmacy. Preferable medications may include (Salzman, 19 82):

Benzodiazepines: Oxazepam and lorazepam (least likely to
accumulate). In patients with insomnia, try relaxation
or exercise first. Only later try flurazepam or the
sedating antihistamines (eg, diphenhydramine and
hydroxyzine).
Tricyclics: Nortriptyline (less cardiotoxicity and hypotension) and desipramine (few anticholinergic effects).
Begin as low as 10-25 mg daily and work up. Test for
glaucoma and prostatic hypertrophy first. Monitor blood
levels.
MAOIs: All have little anticholinergic effect and cardiotoxicity but watch out for hypotension. They are
effective antidepressants, but hypertensive crises are
particularly worrisome in the elderly.
Antipsychotics: Usually choose the more potent, least
sedating types (eg, haloperidol, trifluoperazine), but
be guided by patient's side effects. Thioridazine is
well tolerated in low doses. Be particularly careful
with IM meds - use U-100 insulin syringes to assure a
small dose, if necessary.
Lithium: Toxicity occurs easily (Smith and Helms, 1982) so
keep on a lower maintenance level (eg, .6-.7 meq/l).

GENERAL TREATMENT PRINCIPLES

- Be supportive, respectful, sympathetic, and a "good
  listener." Touch the patient.
- Encourage patients to express themselves (about guilt,
  loneliness, helplessness) and unburden themselves (eg,
  grieve).
- Be directive and reality-oriented. Help in a concrete
  way with problems (eg, who to see about rent assistance,
  calling "Meals-on-Wheels," explanation of Medicare
  benefits). The quality of the patient's current
  environment is probably the single most important factor
  promoting recovery and continued health.
- Strengthen defenses rather than restructure them.
- Encourage self-esteem. Helping patients "review their
  life" (to see it as complete) can be enormously
  beneficial. Reminiscence is adaptive coping behavior
  and helps promote self-esteem.
- Encourage continued interests, friendships, socialization, activities, and self-support. Identify those
  things still done well and keep the patient doing them
  (if they can't fix the meal, maybe they can still set
  the table).
- Be an ongoing presence. Be available - frequent,
  regular, short sessions. Be reachable by telephone.
- Involve and work with the family. Teach them appropriate
  skills and expectations. Anger, frustrations, and
  resentment often develop - help them deal with these
  feelings.

- A psychotherapy group of elderly patients is often very helpful - locate one for the patient.
- Know and use community resources.

REFERENCES

1. Barnes R, Raskind M: Strategies for diagnosing and treating agitation in the aging. Geriatrics 35:111, Apr. 1980.
2. Birren JE, Sloane RB: Handbook of Mental Health and Aging. Englewood Cliffs, NJ, Prentice-Hall, 1980.
3. Blazer DG: Depression in Late Life. St Louis, C.V. Mosby Co., 1982.
4. Brink TL: Geriatric Psychotherapy. New York, Human Sciences Pr, 1979.
5. Brinkman SD, Largen JW: Changes in brain ventricular size with repeated CAT scans in suspected Alzheimer's disease. Am J Psychiat 141:81, 1984.
6. Busse EW, Blazer DG: Handbook of Geriatric Psychiatry. New York, Van Nostrand Reinhold, 1980.
7. Butler RN, Lewis MI: Aging and Mental Health, 2nd ed. Saint Louis, C.V. Mosby Co, 1982.
8. Gurland BJ, Toner JA: Depression in the elderly: a review of recently published studies. Ann Rev Geront and Geriat 3:228, 1982.
9. Katona CLE, Lowe D, Jack RL: Prediction of outcome in psychogeriatric patients. Acta Psychiatr Scand 67:297, 1983.
10. Lipowski ZJ: Transient cognitive disorders (delirium, acute confusional states) in the elderly. Am J Psychiat 140:1426, 1983.
11. Mace NL, Rabins PV: The 36-Hour Day. Baltimore, Johns Hopkins Univ Pr, 1981.
12. Meyers BS, Mei-tal V: Psychiatric reactions during tricyclic treatment of the elderly reconsidered. J Clin Psychopharm 3:1, 1983.
13. Murphy E: The prognosis of depression in old age. Brit J Psychiat 142:111, 1983.
14. Pettinati HM, Bonner KM: Cognitive functioning in depressed geriatric patients with a history of ECT. Am J Psychiat 141:49, 1984.
15. Salzman C: A primer on geriatric psychopharmacology. Am J Psychiat 139:67, 1982.
16. Salzman C, Shader RI, Greenblatt DJ, Harnatz JS: Long v short half-life benzodiazepines in the elderly. Arch Gen Psychiat 40:293, 1983.
17. Smith RE, Helms PM: Adverse effects of lithium therapy in the acutely ill elderly patient. J Clin Psychiat 43, No 3:94, 1982.

18. Verwoerdt A: Clinical Geropsychiatry, 2nd ed. Baltimore, Williams & Wilkins Co, 1981.
19. Yesavage JA, Karasu TB: Psychotherapy with elderly patients. Am J Psychotherapy 36:41, 1982.

Chapter 25

Legal Issues

The interface between psychiatry and law is in flux, partly due to recent patient's rights legislation (based on the constitutional assurance that no person shall be deprived of his liberty without "due process of law"). A psychiatrist's dealings with his patients increasingly are constrained by case law and statute. It is essential that he learn the limits to his independence. Laws can differ markedly from state to state and may change with time - become familiar with those laws that apply to your area.

CIVIL LAW

CIVIL COMMITMENT:

All states permit civil commitment under specific, but differing, criteria:

1. Mental Illness: All states require the presence of a mental illness, but definitions differ. Psychosis usually is included but personality disorder is not. Drug and/or alcohol abuse may be accepted. Mental illness alone is not sufficient for commitment but requires at least one of the following two additional conditions.
2. Dangerousness - to self or others: Most states require the patient to be dangerous but differ in the degree of urgency - an imminent danger (eg, likely to hurt himself in the next 24 hours) vs a relative danger (eg, physically deteriorating through depressive withdrawal). Two major problems with the danger- ousness standard are: (1) psychiatrists are incapable of accurately predicting future dangerous behavior except in the most obvious cases, and (2) it has been uncertain what level of proof the law requires - ie, the traditional lesser civil standard of "clear and convincing evidence" or the more strict criminal

standard of "beyond a reasonable doubt." This latter
issue appears to have been resolved by a recent US
Supreme Court decision (Addington v Texas, 1979)
favoring "clear and convincing evidence."
3. Disabled and in need of treatment: Although diminished
   in number, some states allow commitment solely on the
   grounds that a person is significantly handicapped by
   a mental illness, is in need of treatment, and would
   benefit from that treatment.

Most states also have laws (usually less strict)
allowing the patient to be briefly (1-14 days) held
involuntarily. Committed patients who feel that they are
being held illegally may obtain a hearing by a writ of
habeas corpus.

Much of recent legislation defining these standards
has redressed real past wrongs which occurred when commitment could result merely from a physician's OK, yet recent
controversy has focused on associated losses to the patient
and his family due to his exclusion from treatment because
of complex, criminal-like commitment proceedings. As fewer
patients have been treated involuntarily, some experts have
noted a shift of mental patients from the civil to the
criminal system (Bonovitz and Guy, 1979) - ie, the mental
illness causes them to break a law they ordinarily would
not have broken and they are then arrested. The extent of
this trend has not yet been determined.

An additional impact of the changing commitment laws
has been to require the release of committed patients much
earlier than in the past, resulting in a marked decline in
the size of state mental hospitals. An unfortunate effect
of this deinstitutionalization has been to release large
numbers of marginally functioning persons into communities
ill-equipped to deal with them - with the resultant
formation of "psychiatric ghettos" in some large cities.

Attempts to improve the civil commitment process
continue (eg, the Stone-Roth model - see Monahan et al,
1982).

THE RIGHT TO TREATMENT:

Following the classic Alabama decision of Wyatt v
Stickney (1972), it has become a general standard
(amazingly, it had not been before) that an involuntarily
committed person must receive a level of effective treatment adequate to encourage improvement. This concept was
challenged, reviewed, and supported in another well-known
case - Donaldson v O'Connor (1974). Still uncertain is

what to do with the patient who is unlikely to improve with
<u>any</u> treatment.

THE RIGHT TO REFUSE TREATMENT:

This is currently the most actively contested area of
psychiatric law and the results of the debate remain
uncertain (Mills et al, 1983). Involuntary commitment is
<u>not</u> prima facie evidence that the patient is incompetent to
decide what treatment he is to receive. Federal court
decisions set the tone but conflict: <u>Rennie v Klein</u> (1979)
gives a patient a qualified right to refuse treatment and
creates an appeal process, while <u>Rogers v Okin</u> (1981)
allows absolute refusal but provides for treatment
authorized by a guardian. Presumably the US Supreme Court
ultimately will clarify these discrepancies, but has not
done so yet. Meanwhile, be <u>very</u> cautious (and legal) when
insisting that a patient receive ECT or medication against
his will, even when he appears to need it badly. Know your
local laws. The degree of a physician's liability in
giving treatment to a resisting patient is likely to be
clarified in the next few years.

COMPETENCY:

Psychiatrists are sometimes asked to decide if a
patient is mentally competent to perform specific functions
(eg, make a will, handle his finances, testify in court).
There are rules for some of these decisions - eg, to be
judged competent to make a will, a person must know (1)
that he is making a will, (2) the extent and nature of his
property, and (3) to whom he is leaving his things. To be
found incompetent for one task does not necessarily imply
incompetence for another.

CRIMINAL LAW

COMPETENCY TO STAND TRIAL:

It is held in law that, to receive a fair trial, a
person must be able to understand the nature of his
charges, understand the possible penalties, understand
legal issues and procedures, and work with his attorney and
participate rationally in his own defense. If he can't do
one or more of these, he is "incompetent to stand trial"
and usually is transferred to a treatment facility until
his competency is restored (eg, medication for a
psychosis). Once found competent, the patient is usually
returned to court to stand trial. Recently, some states
have decided that if a patient's competency can't be

restored in a "reasonable length of time" (eg, the length
of time he probably would serve for the crime for which he
has been charged), he must continue treatment in a civil
facility if commitable, or be released. Psychiatrists are
most commonly the experts asked to help the court decide on
competency (the decision is the court's).

CRIMINAL RESPONSIBILITY:

The "not guilty by reason of insanity" plea is much
debated by both the legal and psychiatric professions yet
it continues to be used (infrequently). It is not widely
abused. Part of the general dissatisfaction with this plea
centers on whether psychiatrists (or anyone) can retro-
spectively determine a patient's mental functioning at the
time of a crime. Just as an incompetency decision is
concerned with the patient's mental state at the time of
the trial, a responsibility decision involves the mental
state at the time of the crime. Also in question are the
criteria needed to make that judgment - several different
ones are used in different states:

- The M'Naghten Rule: Did the person not know (1) the
    nature of his act and (2) that it was wrong? This is
    a common test (1/3 of states).
- The Irresistible Impulse Test: Was he acting under an
    "irresistible impulse?" This test is invariably
    combined with other tests.
- The Durham Rule: Was his act the product of "a mental
    disease or defect?"
- The American Law Institute (ALI) Test: Does he have a
    mental disease or defect such that he "lacks
    substantial capacity either to appreciate the
    criminality of his conduct or to conform his conduct
    to the requirements of the law?" This test adds a
    "volitional" standard to the "cognitive" standard of
    the M'Naghten Rule. It is used in approximately 1/2
    of the states and in all federal courts.

If one or more of the above conditions are met, the patient
may be declared "not guilty by reason of insanity" and be
freed of responsibility for his crime. If needing
treatment at that point, he is usually placed in a
psychiatric facility until his mental illness remits or
until he is no longer felt to be a threat to the community
because of mental illness.

Many states and the US Congress have considered
restrictive modifications (or abolition) of the insanity
defense in the wake of the public outcry following John
Hinckley's "not guilty" verdict in his shooting of

President Reagan. The form the insanity defense ultimately will take is not clear (Insanity Defense Work Group, 1983). Leading possibilities appear to be (1) a return to some form of the M'Naghten Rule by eliminating the "volitional" standard, and (2) a guilty but mentally ill verdict (thus, a person first would be judged and sentenced criminally, then treated in prison for his mental illness).

PERSONAL ISSUES

MALPRACTICE:

The risk that a psychiatrist will be successfully sued for malpractice is low but climbing. Most suits involve use of ECT, improper or inadequately informed use of medication, unusual treatments, sexual involvement with patients, and successful patient suicide (suit brought by the patient's family).

CONFIDENTIALITY:

Physicians are ethically obligated to maintain patient confidentiality, except when voluntarily waived by the patient. General knowledge by others of details of a patient's psychiatric treatment or even awareness of psychiatric care can be damaging socially and occupationally to a patient. Unfortunately, legal protection of the physician for maintaining that confidentiality is far from complete. In some cases (eg, Tarasoff v Regents of the University of California (1975), which obligates a therapist to worn a third party threatened harm by the patient), the psychiatrist may be liable if he does not break privacy. In addition, utilization review groups and third-party payers are demanding more privileged information. Some psychiatrists have begun keeping double sets of records - only the "edited" one is released. Become familiar with your own state's laws.

INFORMED CONSENT:

Informed consent should be sought from all patients for all treatments, but formal (ie, written) consent should be obtained for physical procedures (eg, ECT, medication). The patient should be informed about the reasons for the treatment, it's nature, the likelihood of success, the dangers and likelihood of side effects, and any alternative treatments.

A major problem arises if the patient is "incapable of being informed" (eg, due to retardation, OBS, psychosis).

A guardian may need to be appointed whose duty would be to make the decision for the patient.

REFERENCES

1. Abernethy V: Compassion, control, and decisions about competency. Am J Psychiat 141:53, 1984.
2. Bonovitz JC, Guy EB: Impact of restrictive civil commitment procedures on a prison psychiatric service. Am J Psychiat 136:1045, 1979.
3. Halleck SL: Malpractice in psychiatry. Psy Clin N Am 6:567, 1983.
4. Holden C: Insanity defence reexamined. Science 222:994, 1983.
5. Insanity Defense Work Group: American Psychiatric Association statement on the insanity defense. Am J Psychiat 140:681, 1983.
6. Mills MJ, Yesavage JA, Gutheil TG: Continuing case law development in the right to refuse treatment. Am J Psychiat 140:715, 1983.
7. Monahan J, Ruggiero M, Friedlander HD: Stone-Roth model of civil commitment and the California dangerousness standard. Arch Gen Psychiat 39:1267, 1982.
8. Smith SM: Competency. Psy Clin N Am 6:635, 1983.
9. Stone AA: Mental Health and Law: A System in Transition. New York, Jason Aronson Inc, 1976.
10. Wanck B: Two decades of involuntary hospitalization legislation. Am J Psychiat 141:33, 1984.
11. Weiner MF, Shuman DW: The privilege study. Arch Gen Psychiat 40:1027, 1983.
12. Williams PW: New developments in civil commitment of the mentally ill. JAMA 242:2307, 1979.
13. Wulsin LR, Bursztajn H, Gutheil TG: Unexpected clinical features of the Tarasoff decision: the therapeutic alliance and the "duty to warn". Am J Psychiat 140:601, 1983.

Index